Praise for The Fast800 Diet

"The revolutionary new diet by Dr. Michael Mosley, creator of the 5:2 [diet]. It is the most eagerly awaited health book of the year."

—*Daily Mail* (London)

"Dr. Michael Mosley has created a practical and easy approach to losing weight fast and sustainably. It is an essential update of the original 5:2, from the creator of the 5:2!"

—Dr. Giles Yeo, geneticist and weight-loss expert, Cambridge University

"A triumph, providing just the right balance of practical advice, scientific reasoning, and hope."

—Dr. Jack Lewis, broadcaster and neuroscientist

"Dr. Mosley, one of the world's leading writers covering nutrition and health, does it again with a very informative and entertaining book."

—Dr. Valter Longo, director of the Longevity Institute, University of Southern California

ALSO BY DR. MICHAEL MOSLEY

The 8-Week Blood Sugar Diet

The FastDiet

FastExercise

The FastLife

The Clever Gut Diet

Fast Asleep

the fast 800 diet

Discover the Ideal Fasting Formula to Shed Pounds, Fight Disease, and Boost Your Overall Health

DR. MICHAEL MOSLEY

ATRIA PAPERBACK
New York • London • Toronto • Sydney • New Delhi

ATRIA PAPERBACK

An Imprint of Simon & Schuster, Inc.
1230 Avenue of the Americas
New York, NY 10020

For information about special discounts for bulk purchases, please contact Simon & Schuster Special Sales at 1-866-506-1949 or business@simonandschuster.com.

The Simon & Schuster Speakers Bureau can bring authors to your live event. For more information or to book an event contact the Simon & Schuster Speakers Bureau at 1-866-248-3049 or visit our website at www.simonspeakers.com.

Food Photography by Smith & Gilmour
Food Styling by Phil Mundy

Manufactured in the United States of America

3 5 7 9 10 8 6 4 2

Library of Congress Cataloging-in-Publication Data has been applied for.

ISBN 978-1-9821-0689-8
ISBN 978-1-9821-0690-4 (pbk)
ISBN 978-1-9821-0691-1 (ebook)

CONTENTS

INTRODUCTION

In 2012 I wrote a book with journalist Mimi Spencer called *The FastDiet*. In that book we laid out the principles and health benefits of what was then a very novel way of dieting called "intermittent fasting."

Although we mentioned different ways of fasting, we focused on something that I called "the 5:2 approach." Instead of cutting your calories every day, as you would on a standard diet, I suggested it might be easier to cut down to around 600 calories for men, and 500 calories for women, on two days a week, and then eat normally on the other five days.

It was a message that really resonated. *The FastDiet* rapidly became an international bestseller, translated into 40 languages, and the diet was embraced by a wide range of people, including doctors, politicians, celebrities, and Nobel Prize winners. Jimmy Kimmel, the comedian and host of *Jimmy Kimmel Live!*, lost 25 lb on the 5:2, and has kept it off by continuing to cut his calories two days a week. He recently told *Men's Journal* that it makes you appreciate food more.

The actor Benedict Cumberbatch said he did it "for Sherlock."

The National Health Service (NHS) website, which originally described the 5:2 as a "fad diet," now says in its "Top Diets Review" that "sticking to a regimen for two days a week can be more achievable than seven days, so you may be more likely to persevere with this way of eating and successfully lose weight."

It goes on to add, "Two days a week on a restricted diet can lead to greater reductions in body fat, insulin resistance, and other chronic diseases."[1]

From the 5:2 to the 8-Week Blood Sugar Diet

I first became interested in intermittent fasting when I discovered, through a random blood test, that I had type 2 diabetes. The doctor said that I needed to go on medication. This was a nasty shock because my overweight dad had developed diabetes in his fifties and died of diabetes-related illnesses at the relatively young age of 74. I didn't want to go down the same path.

So I set out to find if there was a drug-free way to "cure" my diabetes, and that's when I first heard about the idea of periodically fasting for both weight loss and better general health. It sounded so interesting that I persuaded the BBC to let me make a science documentary about it called *Eat, Fast, Live Longer*, with myself as the guinea pig.

I tested a number of different forms of intermittent fasting before settling on the 5:2. Using that approach, I managed to lose 19.8 lb and get my blood sugars back to normal, without medication.

Then, a few years later, I came across some startling new research being carried out by Professor Roy Taylor, a diabetes specialist at Newcastle University. He told me the main reason I had managed to knock my diabetes on the head was that I had lost a lot of weight, fast. He had done studies showing that, if you lose over 10% of your body weight (which I had), the fat is drained from your liver and pancreas, and your body is restored to its former health.

When we first met, Roy had just started a big trial, hoping to prove that an 800-calorie-a-day rapid weight-loss diet would not only lead to massive weight loss but also help most patients with type 2 diabetes come off all medication and restore their blood sugars to normal.

This was revolutionary stuff, as most doctors believe that type 2 diabetes is incurable and the only way to treat it is with drugs.

I became so convinced by Roy's research that, with his help, I wrote a second book, *The 8-Week Blood Sugar Diet*. In this book, which is aimed at people with type 2 diabetes and prediabetes (those whose blood sugars are raised but not yet in the diabetic range), I described how to follow a rapid weight-loss program, cutting your calorie intake to 800 a day. This book also became an international bestseller, and thousands of people who followed the program have managed to get their blood sugars back under control without medication. Doctors, nurses, and diabetes specialists now recommend the book in clinical practice. My wife, Clare, is a GP and has been using this approach to transform the lives of hundreds of her patients. One patient lost so much weight Clare didn't recognize him! She is passionate about the power of food to change lives and created the recipes for this book.

So what's new?

Well, first and foremost, there's some startling new science. In the years since writing *The FastDiet* and *The 8-Week Blood Sugar Diet*, I have collected lots of research and data on every aspect of intermittent fasting.

Scientific studies take a long time. The results of Professor Taylor's big diabetes trial—started in 2014—were finally published in 2018 and I'm delighted to say that they were even better than hoped (see Chapter 4). More recently, two other big studies have shown the benefits of following a rapid weight-loss diet based on 800 calories a day, even if you don't have diabetes. A number of new studies have also been done on the wider health benefits of the 5:2.

Which is why, six years on, I have decided to completely update my first two books and to combine the best elements of the latest research in one easy-to-follow program. I've called this new program the Fast800. It still incorporates the 5:2, but is based on, among other things, more manageable 800-calorie fast days. It is designed to provide a simple, effective way to shed fat and set yourself up for a healthier future.

The Fast800

There are various ways you can do the Fast800, and in Chapter 7 I'm going to give you a number of options so that you can tailor the program to your needs, goals, and motivation.

What all these options have in common is that they are based on 800-calorie fast days. That's because 800 is the magic number when it comes to successful dieting—it's high enough to be manageable and sustainable but low enough to trigger a range of desirable metabolic changes.

The choice you have to make, after reading the first part of this book, is how intensively you want to do the program—i.e., how many 800-calorie days to include each week from the start, and how to adjust these as you progress.

For rapid weight loss, as long as it is safe for you to do it (see page 85), 800 calories a day, every day, is what you should be aiming at. This is a regimen that has been shown to be safely sustainable for weeks and months. You might want to take this approach if you have a lot of weight to lose; if you are in a hurry; if you have prediabetes or type 2 diabetes; if you have a fatty liver; if you want to kick your weight-loss journey off with a bang; or perhaps because you have hit a weight-loss plateau.

On 800 calories a day you can expect to lose up to 11 lb after two weeks, 19.8 lb after four weeks, and 30.8 lb after eight weeks, most of which will be fat. Rapid weight loss is often described as "crash dieting" but I want to show you how, done properly, it can be safely used.

However, not everyone can or will want to stick to 800 calories a day for long. So after a few weeks of rapid weight loss, I suggest you consider switching to what I'm calling the "New 5:2." The calorie amounts I came up with for the original FastDiet—500–600 calories twice a week—were based on some human studies, but mainly on animal research. Effective though it is, some people found this approach a bit too tough. So I now recommend cutting to 800 calories twice a week. Will you still lose weight, fast? Yes, particularly if you start with the rapid weight-loss approach, and then move to the New 5:2.

A low-carbohydrate Mediterranean diet

The menus at the back of this book offer plenty of filling and tasty recipes for making up 800-calorie days. They are all based on a low-carb, high-protein Mediterranean-style approach.

The reason I am so keen on this way of eating is that it will help you maintain your muscle mass and stop your metabolic rate from crashing as you lose weight. This means you will find it much easier to keep the weight off, long term. It is also a way of eating that doesn't demand you cut out whole food groups, so I believe it is far more sustainable.

Above all, with the Fast800, I want you to feel free to experiment. We all have different needs and different demands in our lives. My approach is based on the latest science but is also a very pragmatic one. In the end, the best diet is the one you can stick to and which fits best in your life.

Other elements of the Fast800 program

Besides busting a lot of commonly held myths about dieting and weight gain, and bringing you up to date with the latest research, I want to introduce you to a relatively new form of intermittent fasting called Time Restricted Eating (TRE).

TRE has taken the internet by storm, particularly among the body-conscious under-30s. It involves eating all your calories within a relatively narrow time window each day, usually 8 to 12 hours. This extends the length of your normal overnight fast (the time when you are asleep and not eating) and gives your body an opportunity to burn fat and do essential repairs.

TRE is not an alternative to the 5:2; rather, it complements it. I will be going into TRE in some detail in Chapter 2.

I am also going to be writing about the importance of ketosis—that is, persuading your body to switch from using sugars to burning fats in the form of ketone bodies to obtain fuel. This is key to the success of intermittent fasting. It also turns out to be surprisingly good for the body and the brain. But it has to be done the right way.

Why losing weight is about more than vanity

There are good reasons for doing intermittent fasting that go beyond weight loss (and I cover them later in the book), but the people who will benefit most are likely to be those who are currently overweight, particularly those who are carrying too much weight around the middle (i.e., internal, visceral fat).

There is, understandably, a lot of skepticism about

dieting on the grounds that they never work and, anyway, isn't losing weight just about vanity?

There are certainly plenty of ineffective diets out there—I hope to persuade you that this one is different. As for vanity, well, there is nothing wrong with wanting to look better, but the real purpose of the Fast800 is to make you healthier. Even relatively modest changes can make a big difference.

Studies have shown that if you are overweight or obese, losing 5% of your body weight will:

- Reduce your blood pressure and levels of blood fats (triglycerides), which in turn will significantly cut your risk of having a heart attack or stroke.
- Lower your risk of getting cancer. Carrying too much fat in the body leads to the release of hormones and inflammatory agents that boost cancer. According to Cancer Research UK, many cancers are linked to being overweight or obese, including two of the most common: breast and bowel cancer.
- Sleep better. If you are anything like me, when you put on weight it not only goes around your belly, but also around your neck. A fat neck means you are more likely to snore (which will keep your partner awake), and also far more likely to develop obstructive sleep apnea, a disorder that causes people to stop breathing while sleeping. A

2014 study found that people who lost 5% or more of their body weight got about 20 minutes more sleep, and it was better-quality sleep.

- Cut your risk of developing type 2 diabetes. In one big study, people with prediabetes (raised blood sugars, not yet in the diabetic range) who lost over 5% of their body weight were 58% less likely to develop type 2 diabetes than those who didn't.

- Boost your sex drive. Not just because you may feel more desirable but also because of hormonal changes and improved blood flow to the sex organs.

Supersize Me

I normally only recommend things that I have tried myself, because that way I discover just how practical (or not) my suggestions really are.

When I began researching this book, I wondered what would happen if I let myself go, put on weight, then tried to take it off again, using the Fast800 approach.

So, that's what I did. I didn't go crazy, but I did begin to eat more toast and pasta, and have more snacks. Initially, it didn't make much difference. My body was clearly happy with my new, lower weight and it wasn't keen to let me balloon. But, after a month or so, the weight began to creep upward. It took me nearly four months to put on 14 lb and by then my blood sugars were almost back in the diabetic range, my blood pressure had gone up into the red zone, my sleep was terrible, and I felt sluggish and moody. If you want to see what I looked like, visit thefast800.com.

My wife, Clare, told me it was time to stop. So I put myself on the Fast800—with dramatic results (see page 162).

My background

I trained as a medical doctor in London but I have spent many years as a science journalist, working for newspapers and on television. I spend my professional life trying to make sense of complex and often conflicting health claims.

As a result, I am in regular contact with leading doctors, weight-loss specialists, and nutritional researchers from all around the world. I have collaborated with some of these scientists to produce original research, particularly in the area of food and health.

Everything I write is based on cutting-edge science—indeed this book is only possible because so many hard-working scientists have been willing to give me the time to share their latest findings—and as you will see at the back of the book there are lots of references to scientific studies. You don't have to read them, but they are there if you want to see for yourself the basis of my claims.

For those of you who are confused as to why there are so many conflicting health claims in the media, I have also included, at the back, a section on levels of "proof" (see page 264). I explain what a randomized controlled study is and why it is a more reliable form of evidence than government advice, animal studies, or case-controlled studies.

In addition, you will find, peppered throughout this book, case studies and stories from people who have contacted me to share tips and say how they are getting on. I have found it incredibly helpful to have a website with an active community who not only support each other, but also give regular feedback on how they are doing.

We are social animals and the best way to lose weight and develop better habits is by engaging with others. The evidence is strong that the more support you have, the more likely you are to succeed, so we also run an interactive online program at thefast800.com, providing advice, recipes, meal plans, and tracking options. Do come and join in.

1

WHY WE PUT ON WEIGHT

If you want to slim down it is worth understanding why we get fat in the first place. The obvious answer, "because we eat too much and don't do enough exercise," is too simplistic. It's like going to a tennis coach to improve your game and being told that all you need to do is "win more points than your opponent." True, but not useful.

So why has there been such an explosion in obesity, worldwide, over the last 40 years?

There are plenty of plausible explanations, including increased anxiety, stress, poor sleep, and becoming less active, but top of my list is more snacking and the fact that we are eating lots more junk food—not just more cola, cake, and candy, but refined carbs, up by a whopping 20% since 1980.[2] These foods are packed with calories and are highly addictive (see page 29). Bursting with sugar and processed fats, they play havoc with our hormones, and one hormone in particular: insulin.

Carbs and insulin

The thing about carbs, particularly the rapidly digestible carbs you find in junk food, but also in white rice and most breads, is that they are swiftly broken down in your gut to release a flood of sugar into your blood. The result is instant energy and a brief feel-good sugar "high." But having lots of sugar in your blood is bad for your body because it damages blood vessels and nerves.

So your pancreas responds by releasing a hormone called insulin. Insulin's main job is to quickly bring high blood-sugar levels back down to normal, and it does this by helping energy-hungry cells, such as those in your muscles and your brain, to take up the sugar.

But if you're constantly snacking and doing very little to burn the calories off, your body will become less and less sensitive to insulin. So, your pancreas has to work harder to produce more and more insulin. It's like shouting at kids. The more you shout, the less attention they pay.

Two bad things now happen:

1. Your fat cells become large and inflamed, as your body tries to cram more and more energy into them. At some point you exceed your "personal fat threshold." There is no space left to store fat safely, so it begins to overflow into your internal organs, such as your liver. This is

how the French make foie gras, their famous liver pâté. They feed geese so much starchy corn that their livers are soon bursting with fat.

This "visceral" fat—which also infiltrates your pancreas and wraps itself around your heart—is much more dangerous than fat on your buttocks or thighs. It leads to something known as metabolic syndrome, which in turn leads to heart disease, diabetes, and dementia. If you want to see what it looks like, visit thefast800.com, where there is an image of what my insides looked like before I lost weight. Not for the squeamish.

2. Despite carrying around too much fat, you still feel hungry *all the time*. That's because you now have high insulin levels, which encourage continuous fat storage. Which means there's less fuel around to keep the rest of your body going.

It's as if you're constantly pouring money into your bank account, and then finding it incredibly hard to get it out again. You have money, but you just can't get at it. High levels of insulin prevent your body from accessing and burning its own energy supply.

So, despite the fact that you are carrying around lots of energy in the form of fat, your muscles and your brain can't easily access it. Deprived of fuel, your brain tells you to eat more. So you do. But because your high insulin levels are encouraging fat storage, you get fatter while staying hungry.

In other words, if you have a weight problem it may not be because you lack willpower or you're greedy. It is more likely that, like one in three Americans, you are insulin-resistant and therefore have too much insulin washing around in your blood.

Does this sound crazy? What I'm describing is based on the work of some of the world's leading metabolic specialists.

Dr. Robert Lustig, a renowned pediatric endocrinologist who has treated thousands of overweight children, points out in his excellent book *Fat Chance*, that understanding insulin is crucial to understanding obesity. "Insulin shunts sugar to fat. It makes your fat cells grow. The more insulin, the more fat."

Dr. Lustig blames the modern diet, rich in sugar and refined carbs, for pumping up our insulin levels, a claim supported by many other leading obesity experts, including Dr. David Ludwig, a pediatrician from Harvard Medical School, and Dr. Mark Friedman, head of the Nutrition Science Initiative in San Diego.

As Dr. Ludwig and Dr. Friedman have put it: "The increasing amount and processing of carbohydrates in the American diet has increased insulin levels, put fat cells into storage overdrive, and elicited obesity-promoting biological responses in a large number of people. High consumption of refined carbohydrates—chips, crackers, cakes, soft drinks, sugary breakfast cereals, and even white rice and bread—has increased body weights throughout the population."[3]

Other damaging effects of raised insulin

If you are insulin-resistant and your body is forced to go on producing lots of insulin, this will not only keep you hungry, it will contribute to many other diseases. It will increase your risk of developing dementia, breast and bowel cancer, contribute to high blood pressure, and raise your cholesterol levels. In women, raised insulin levels lead to acne, mood swings, excess hair growth, irregular periods (polycystic ovaries), and infertility.

The good news is that, if you change what you eat and lose weight, your insulin levels will come down. Cassie, a nurse with type 2 diabetes who lost 44 lb doing the 8-Week Blood Sugar Diet—the key tenets of which are incorporated into the Fast800 approach—was not only able to come off all medication but soon became pregnant, after many years of trying, with twins!

"You have not only freed me from food and put me back in charge of my life, but helped me make a miracle possible—which I thought would never happen."

The rise and rise of junk food

The fact that we now eat so many refined and sugary carbs, and eat them so often, isn't an accident. It was an unintended consequence of the low-fat campaign, the biggest and arguably the most disastrous public health experiment in history.

It all began in 1957, the year I was born, when the hugely influential American Heart Association decided to mount a campaign aimed at reducing fat consumption. They weren't, initially, targeting bellies; they were more concerned about hearts. They believed that saturated fat caused heart disease, so it was out with the steak, butter, and cheese; in with the pasta, rice, potatoes, and vegetables.

Or at least that was the plan.

Backed by millions of dollars of government money, the low-fat campaign certainly had an effect. Over the next few decades, Americans cut their consumption of animal fats, such as milk, butter, and cream, by as much as 20%.[4] They didn't, however, replace those fats with healthy fruits and vegetables. Instead, people ate more and more processed foods, which were being heavily promoted by the food industry as "low-fat" or "fat-free." Under the pretense of making food "healthier," the manufacturers stuffed their products with processed vegetable oils (such as margarine) and cheap, sugary carbs. And, as consumption of dairy fats went down and that of sugary carbs went up, obesity rates began to soar.

By the 1980s, when I went to medical school, fat was firmly established as something you had to avoid. Eating fat made you fat. Eating fat, particularly saturated fat, would clog your arteries as surely as pouring fat down a drain will block it.

Although I was slim and I did a lot of exercise, I also ate quite a lot of saturated fat, in the form of milk, meat, and butter. I have a family history of heart disease and strokes and my father was a recently diagnosed diabetic. It was plainly time to act.

Zealously, I persuaded my overweight father to go on a low-fat diet (it didn't work) and harangued my mother until she switched from butter to margarine. Eggs were replaced by cereal for breakfast. Coffee came with a dash of skim milk. Yogurt was always low-fat.

So did I become healthier? Well, no. Over the next few decades I put on about 28 lb, my body fat went up to a paunchy 28%, my cholesterol soared, and I became a type 2 diabetic.

The trouble was that, although I was eating less fat, I was now eating far more carbs. If I had switched to eating lots of healthy, complex carbs that are rich in fiber, such as vegetables and whole grains, then I would probably have been fine. Instead, I was doing what I was told, which was to pile my plate with a lot of starchy carbs such as bread, rice, and potatoes.

What I didn't understand—because they don't teach you much, if anything, about nutrition at medical school—was the effect these foods were having on my body. Eating a boiled potato will push your blood sugars up as quickly as eating a tablespoon of sugar (I've tried it!). Ironically, if you eat the potato with fat, such as cheese or butter, the fat will slow absorption and the blood-sugar peak will be slower and less extreme.

Nor had I appreciated that carbs, particularly refined carbs, are so much less satiating than fat or protein. You have a bowl of cereal for breakfast and a few hours later you are hungry. So you have a snack. On my high-carb diet, I was constantly hungry, so I was snacking all the time. And that was keeping my overworked pancreas busy pumping out insulin—which, as we have seen above, was making me fatter and fatter.

Why snacking makes us fat

People used to believe in the quaint idea of "not eating between meals." In the 1970s, before the modern obesity crisis, adults would average four and a half hours between meals, while children would be expected to last about four hours. Like flared trousers, those times are long gone. Now the average window between meals is down to three and a half hours for adults and three hours for children, and that doesn't include all the drinks and nibbles.

The idea, which has come to dominate, is that "eating little and often" is a good thing. This idea was driven by snack manufacturers and it was and, incredibly, still is supported by some dieticians. The argument goes that it is better to eat lots of small meals—anything up to six a day (i.e., breakfast, lunch, and supper along with mid-morning, afternoon, and bedtime snacks)—because that way we are less likely to get hungry and gorge on high-fat junk. That's the theory. In the real world, people do the opposite.

Compared to 30 years ago, not only do we eat around 180 calories a day more in snacks—much of it in the form of milky, sweetened drinks and smoothies—but also more when it comes to our regular meals, an average of 120 extra calories a day. In other words, the more we snack, the more we eat overall.

Eating throughout the day, from when we first wake to that little treat last thing at night, is now so normal that it is almost shocking to suggest doing the absolute opposite. In other words, fasting. More on that in the next chapter.

Food addiction

The modern obesity epidemic wasn't triggered by a collective breakdown in willpower in the late 1970s. It happened because food manufacturers have found more and more ingenious ways to make us buy their products. Like the tobacco industry, they know how to hook and hold their customers.

Junk food is clearly not addictive in the same way that cocaine is, but it shares some of its qualities. The pleasure you get from it is normally very short-lived. It is about compulsion. We eat junk food knowing it is bad for us. We do it because we can't stop ourselves. The purveyors of junk food like to claim that it's okay to have "a little bit of everything" or "everything in moderation." You wouldn't say that about arsenic.

I love chocolate, particularly milk chocolate. My cravings for chocolate have nothing to do with hunger. There are times when I can be ravenously hungry, be in a supermarket, and find it easy to walk past the prominently displayed racks of chocolate. There are other times, particularly late at night, when I find myself prowling around our kitchen, looking in cupboards for the stash of chocolate that I think Clare may have left somewhere.

I have bought a bar of chocolate in a motorway service station, thrown it into the back seat to stop myself wolfing it down, then pulled into the next service station to eat it. I have broken up a chocolate bar and thrown it in a bin and then, minutes later, started to root around in that bin. A particularly low point was when I ate my six-year-old daughter's Easter egg.

Don't tell me this behavior is normal.

These cravings are strongest late at night, when I am tired, but also when I am stressed, upset, or simply bored. I have tried to wean myself onto dark chocolate, but that doesn't fulfill the same emotional needs. I am a chocaholic and suspect I will always be.

Which are the most addictive foods and why?

Some people claim that sugar is addictive, but even a moment's thought will show you that can't be true. I love sweet treats but even I don't routinely bury my face in a bowl of sugar.

I recently tried eating a small bowl of sugar and began to gag halfway through the first tablespoon. It is not an experience I want to repeat.

So what is it that so many addictive foods have in common?

In 2015 researchers from the University of Michigan decided to find out.[5] They got 120 students, offered them a choice of 35 different foods, and asked them to fill in the Yale Food Addiction Scale, a measure of how addictive you find a particular food. The foods were then ranked from 1 to 35 by the students.

Not surprisingly, top of the list of "most addictive foods" was chocolate, followed by ice cream, French fries, pizza, cookies, chips, cake, buttered popcorn, and cheeseburgers.

Somewhere in the middle were cheese, bacon, and nuts, while at the bottom were salmon, brown rice, cucumber, and broccoli.

When you look at the list below, what strikes you? The first thing is that the highly addictive foods are also highly processed foods, designed to be absorbed very rapidly and give your brain an almost immediate dopamine (the reward hormone) rush. In addition, they are the sort of foods that are heavily advertised, particularly to children.

But the thing that really sets them apart is that they are a mixture of fats and carbs. And not any old mixture. Broadly speaking, whether it is chocolate or chips, cake or cheeseburger, they are all made up of roughly 1g fat to 2g carbs. It is a ratio that we seem to find particularly irresistible.

The 2:1 ratio

Milk chocolate, per 100g	30g fat	58g carbs	534 calories
Ice cream, per 100g	12g fat	24g carbs	200 calories
French fries, per 100g	15g fat	32g carbs	270 calories
Pepperoni pizza, per 100g	10g fat	30g carbs	266 calories
Chips, per 100g	30g fat	50g carbs	536 calories
Sponge cake	26g fat	52g carbs	460 calories
Buttered popcorn	30g fat	56g carbs	546 calories
Cheeseburger	14g fat	30g carbs	303 calories

As you can see, it is not an exact 2:1 ratio for all these foods, but it is pretty close. Why should that be? Well, one reason we find this particular ratio so appealing may be that we found it in the first food we ever consumed, breast milk. A 3.3 oz serving of human breast milk contains around 4g fat and 8g carbs, making it surprisingly sweet.

In fact, milk is one of the very few natural foods that contains high amounts of fat and carbs all mixed together. Meat is high in fat and protein, but very low in carbs, while vegetables can contain lots of carbs but not much fat.

We aren't the only animal who just can't say "no" to this killer combination. Lab rats, given access to lots of fat alone or carbs alone, will eat just enough to maintain a steady body weight. But if you give them unrestricted access to foods rich in both fats and carbohydrates, they will gorge and gorge until they are almost spherical.

Food manufacturers, of course, are well aware of our vulnerabilities and exploit them to sell us their products. Knowing this may not change your food compulsions, but at least it will help you understand why you go on craving food that is bad for you and may help you fight back. Ever since I told my kids some of the things that "Big Food" has done to get us hooked, they have been less enthusiastic about going to places like McDonald's.

Are you addicted to a particular food?

Try this short quiz to see how addicted you are to a particular food. More than three "yes" answers and you may be in trouble. I try to avoid ice cream and chips because I know that when I start, I find it hard to stop, but the only food on the "addictive" list I have real problems with is chocolate.

Thinking about chocolate, I said "yes" to questions 1, 2, 3, 4, 7, 9, and 10. Which gives me a score of 7. There is no other food I can think of where I would score more than 2.

1. When I start eating this food, I can't stop and end up eating much more than I intended.
2. I keep on eating this food even when I am no longer hungry.
3. I eat to the point where I feel physically ill.
4. I find myself craving this food when I'm stressed.
5. If it isn't in the house, I will get in the car and drive to the nearest shop that sells it.
6. I use this food to make myself feel better.
7. I hide this food so even those close to me don't know how much of it I eat.
8. Eating it causes anxiety and feelings of self-loathing and guilt.
9. Although I no longer get much pleasure from eating it, I keep on doing so.
10. I have tried to give this food up but failed.

Add up your "yes" answers. The more you gave the answer yes, the more hooked on carbs you are.

I will be writing more about food cravings and how to beat them in Chapter 7.

In summary:

- The reason we are snacking more and eating more junk foods is no accident: junk food is packed with fat, sugar, and salt. It has been designed to make us crave it.
- Eating lots of refined carbs—in the form of white bread, rice, and pasta, as well as junk food—will keep your pancreas pumping out insulin.
- High insulin levels keep us hungry, which in turn makes us snack more.
- If you follow my program, you will not only lose weight but also bring your insulin levels down. You won't feel as hungry and you will see lots of other improvements.

2

INTERMITTENT FASTING COMES OF AGE

The program I am recommending in this book is based on numerous scientific studies, feedback from hundreds of successful intermittent fasters, and from talking to lots of weight-loss specialists. It is designed to achieve the maximum benefit in the most achievable way. But everyone is different, so I want you to feel free to experiment with the approach or approaches that work best for you.

Before you start, I also want you to understand what intermittent fasting has to offer, not just for weight loss but for health issues such as reducing inflammation, risk of heart disease, improving gut health, and much more. So, in this chapter I am going to do a deep dive into the science behind the different forms of intermittent fasting, assessing their strengths and weaknesses.

Meet the CRONies

As I mentioned in the introduction, intermittent fasting is now very popular. But when I set out to explore this approach to eating back in 2012, it was seen as both eccentric and dangerous. Public interest had yet to take off and there were relatively few human studies. Not many celebs were into it. In fact, most of those who practiced fasting, intermittent or otherwise, were either doing it for religious reasons, or were body builders or New Agers. Or CRONies (Calorie Restrictors on Optimal Nutrition).

CRONies—there are an estimated 100,000 of them worldwide—practice something called long-term calorie restriction (CR). This involves drastically cutting back your calories every day—forever—in the hope that this will extend your life.

It doesn't sound much fun; in fact, it sounds a lot like chronic starvation or an eating disorder. But an important difference is that, although CRONies are on a low-calorie diet, they are careful to get all the essential vitamins, minerals, and nutrients. They are eating healthily, just not very much.

CRONies, who are mainly men, typically live on a diet of around 1,600 calories a day, every day. That is about two thirds of the amount that an average man would eat.

Curious as to why anyone would want to do that, I

managed, via the CR society website,[6] to track down a CRONie called Dave. Dave, who had been calorie restricting for more than two decades, also lives conveniently close to me in southern England. Even better, he's the same age as I am, to within a few weeks.

Dave began calorie restricting when he was in his early thirties. Why? "I didn't pay much attention to my diet or drinking when I was a student," he told me. "I'd eat and drink anything and everything. But in about 1988 there was a lot of publicity about heart disease and how it could be a killer in your forties and fifties and I started to seriously adjust my diet."

He began by cutting out chocolate and wheat, which made him feel better. "I'd suffered from migraines and suddenly they stopped. Then I read the *120-Year Diet Book* by Roy Walford, the founding father of the calorie restriction diet, and I decided to cut my calories down to 1,600."

Dr. Roy Walford was one of the early champions of calorie restriction. As a research scientist he had shown that you can really extend a mouse's life by keeping it on a low-calorie diet. He had also taken part in a slightly crazy human experiment called Biosphere 2, which involved living with a group of other volunteers in a sealed building in the Arizona desert. The point of this experiment was to prepare humans to live on another planet. To do this, the volunteers cut themselves off from the outside world, living only on the food they could grow, and recycling water and air.

Walford persuaded everyone to live on a low-calorie diet for most of the two years they were inside. Not surprisingly, they lost a lot of weight, and Walford declared it a huge success. However, despite claiming that following a CR lifestyle would help you live healthily to 120, Walford went on to die at the unremarkable age of 79. Will Dave and his fellow CRONies fare better?

The battle of the bodies

To see if the CR lifestyle was doing Dave any good, we agreed to compare bodies. So we had a full medical. Dave, who is an inch shorter than me, was nearly 44 lb lighter. He had a body fat of just 8% (mine, at the time, was 26%) and he had the blood pressure of a 20-year-old. His arteries were clear and his hearing, balance, and sense of touch were far better than mine.

But the most revealing moment came when we visited a leading plastic surgeon and without telling him why, asked him to estimate our ages. The surgeon accurately and brutally guessed that I was in my fifties, "because of your jowly bits." He decided that Dave was 20 years younger than me, "because his skin is almost wrinkle-free and has far more elasticity than yours."

So Dave is looking remarkably good for his age,

albeit a bit skinny, and his body seems to be in fine shape. We will have to wait another few decades to know whether he will really live longer than the rest of us. But the latest evidence from animals suggests they just might.

Fasting lemurs live longer

We've known since the 1930s that you can extend the life of a mouse by restricting what it eats, but it wasn't until recently that we could be sure it would work with an animal that was more like us.

In June 2018 scientists published the results of a really long-term study on the mouse lemur.[7] Despite the name, mouse lemurs have nothing to do with mice. They are primates, which means they are part of the same extended family as monkeys and humans. They are relatively short-lived (which is convenient if you are studying aging) and their body chemistry is similar to ours.

To do their experiment, researchers from the National Institute of Aging took a large group of mouse lemurs and divided them into two groups. The groups were brought up in similar conditions and on the same healthy foods. The only difference was that one group, from early adulthood, was made to live on 30% fewer calories than the other group (the control group).

So what happened? Well, as the years went by the differences became more and more obvious. The calorie-restricted lemurs stayed young-looking and glossy. They had much lower rates of cancer and diabetes, and tests on their mental abilities showed they remained on the ball. Brain scans also revealed that they had preserved a lot more white matter, the neuronal fibers that connect different areas of the brain, than the lemurs on a normal diet.

Most impressive of all, they lived on average 50% longer than their better-fed cousins. This is reasonably convincing evidence that calorie restriction really can extend the life of an animal like us. Almost a third of the calorie-restricted animals were still alive when the last animal in the control group died.

More manageable forms of fasting

It may extend your life, but becoming a CRONie is not something most of us aspire to. I want the benefits of calorie restriction without the drawbacks. And that's why I am so excited about intermittent fasting. Cutting your calories for short periods of time, or restricting *when* you eat your calories, seems to offer many of the benefits of long-term calorie restriction. And it is an awful lot easier and far more convenient.

In this chapter I am going to bring you up to date

with the latest science behind three of the most popular forms of intermittent fasting, which are:

- Periodic fasting (where, once every few months, you cut your food down for five days in a row).
- The 5:2 approach (where you restrict your calories for two days a week).
- Time Restricted Eating (where you restrict your eating to a narrow time window).

Each of these forms of intermittent fasting provides different health benefits. And the great thing is they are not mutually exclusive. Let's look at each of them in turn.

1. PERIODIC FASTING

Professor Valter Longo, director of the University of Southern California's Longevity Institute, is one of the world's leading experts on the science of human aging. Therefore, he was also one of the first scientists I went to in search of answers as to what exactly fasting is, how it works, and why it is so important for human health.

Valter—tall, slim, and aging well—is a great advertisement for his own research. Born in Italy in 1967, he looks a good 10 years younger than his real age.

Valter believes passionately in using the power of fasting to delay aging and prevent the onset of chronic diseases like cancer, heart disease, and diabetes. He has dedicated his life to understanding the mechanisms by which that happens. And the good news is he thinks we now have a pretty good understanding of why aging happens and how to delay it. Even better, you don't have to give up eating well or become a skinny CRONie to live a long and healthy life. So why is fasting, as Valter once said to me, one of the most powerful things you can do?

Autophagy

The list of things that fasting does to your body is long and complex, but one of the more striking benefits comes from activating a process within the body called "autophagy," which literally means "self-eat." Autophagy is an entirely natural process where dead, diseased, or worn-out cells are broken down and gobbled up.

Think of your body as a bit like a car. When it's new, it's bright and shiny and everything works. But as time goes by, bits get worn out and some parts start to rust. If you insist on driving it around continuously at high speed, then it will, eventually, fall apart.

To keep your car going for as long as possible you need to take it to a garage so that mechanics can remove and replace worn-out parts and spruce it up. An obvious truth is you can't repair your car and drive it hard, all at the same time.

The same is true of us. Just as we need sleep, we also need time off from constant eating if we are to turn on the repair genes that keep us in good shape. It is only when we are not eating or drinking anything with calories in it that our bodies can begin this process of repair.

Autophagy is triggered by fasting, and becomes more intense as time goes by. It stops once you eat.

Regeneration

Fasting triggers autophagy, which means your body is able to clear away the junk and the debris, i.e., old cells. But what happens when you start to eat? Is all the good you've done then undone?

In 2014 Valter and his colleagues did an experiment to find out.[8] They took a group of mice and made them fast for two days at a time, over a period of several months. One of the first things that happened was that their white blood cell count started to fall. This, as Valter explained, was an expected and healthy response. "When you fast, your system tries to save energy, and one of the things it does is recycle a lot of the immune cells that are not needed, especially those that are old or damaged."

But what happened when the mice were allowed to feed after their fast? Their bodies immediately responded with the creation of new, more active white cells.

"We could not have predicted," Valter said, "that fasting would have such a remarkable effect."

It seems that fasting, by triggering autophagy, also creates space for new cells to grow. It's like a forest fire that burns away the old undergrowth, making space for new plants and trees.

Fasting, followed by feeding, gives the "okay" for the body to go ahead and begin creating new cells. So if your immune system is not as effective as it once was (either because you are older or because you have had a medical treatment, such as chemotherapy), then short periods of fasting may help regenerate it.

Jenni's story

Jenni Russell, a British journalist, read Valter's research with great interest. For more than 20 years she had suffered from a serious autoimmune condition that was wrecking her life.

"It often left me sleeping for 12 hours a day," she wrote in her column in the *London Times*, "and sometimes kept me in bed for months at a time."[9]

She was kept going by powerful and expensive immune-suppressing drugs, but these made her feel dreadful, and she was warned she would never be able to live without them.

So when she came across Valter's research showing that short-term fasting could reprogram a faulty immune system, she decided she would give it a go.

"I had nothing to lose by trying it, except my temper and a little weight. I started the first fast on a boat journey on a stormy sea. It was made a lot easier by the fact that I'd lost my appetite anyway, and that I wasn't required to do anything except lie in a bunk and read."

She decided to do her fast the Cossack way. Just water and tea (black, green, or mint). "I got cross, hungry, and despondent, and gave up just before the end of Day 3. Waste of time, I thought."

But then, on the fourth day, she woke up feeling better than she had for years.

Still skeptical, but curious, she tried doing another short fast a few weeks later. "This time," she wrote, "every symptom vanished. I could not believe what had happened. I went on fasting every few weeks, just to be sure, but three and a half years later, not one of my symptoms has reccurred. I take no drugs. I have my life back."

Flipping the metabolic switch

Under Valter's guidance, and as part of a BBC science program I made back in 2012 (*Eat, Fast, Live Longer*),

I did a fairly draconian four-day fast myself. As well as unlimited water and black tea, I decided to allow myself a small daily snack, in the shape of 25 calories of miso soup. I came to love that miso soup.

I'd been warned that the first few days might be tough, but after that I would start feeling the effects of a rush of what Valter termed "well-being chemicals."

I got myself weighed, had some blood taken, and then, on a warm Monday evening, I had a last supper of steak, fries, and salad washed down with beer.

During the first 24 hours of a fast, big changes go on inside your body. Within a few hours, the sugar (glucose) circulating in your blood begins to fall. If it's not replaced by food the body turns for energy to a stable form of glucose that is stored in your muscles and liver: glycogen.

Once stores of glycogen begin to run low (10–12 hours after your last meal), your body goes through a remarkable change. It switches over into fat-burning mode. It's called "flipping the metabolic switch." A bit like a hybrid car flipping from using electricity to using petrol when the batteries begin to run low.

When this happens, fat is released from your fat stores and converted by your body into fatty acids and substances called ketone bodies. Like most of your body, your brain will happily use these ketone bodies as a source of energy. In many ways your brain runs better on ketones than on glucose (see page 56).

The first two days of a fast can be uncomfortable, particularly if you have never done anything like it before. That's because your body and brain are having to cope with managing this switch from using glucose to using ketones. If you are not accustomed to it (which most people aren't) you can get headaches, feel exhausted, and may find it hard to sleep.

The biggest problem I had with fasting is hard to put into words; it was sometimes just feeling "uncomfortable." I can't really describe it more accurately than that. I didn't feel faint; I just felt out of place.

I did, occasionally, feel hungry, but most of the time I was surprisingly cheerful. By Day 3, the feel-good hormones had come to my rescue.

By Friday, Day 4, it was over. That afternoon I had myself tested and discovered I had lost 3 lb of body weight, most of which was fat. I was also delighted to discover that my blood levels of IGF-1 (insulin-like growth factor 1), which are a measure of cancer risk, had almost halved.

Periodic fasting and cancer

I was expecting to lose weight on a four-day, liquid-only fast, but I was surprised to see such a dramatic fall in my IGF-1 levels in such a short time.

But this didn't surprise Valter. He has evidence that

regular bouts of short-term fasting can not only reduce your risk of getting a variety of cancers, but may also be used to enhance the effects of chemotherapy should you need treatment for cancer.

How? The thing about normal human cells is that when you cut off their food supply they go into what Valter calls "a highly protected nongrowth mode." In other words, they hunker down and wait for better times.

Cancer cells are different. Even when you are fasting, they keep growing out of control. And this makes them vulnerable to chemo.

Imagine you have cancer and are about to have a course of chemotherapy, which works by killing rapidly dividing cells. The side effects of chemo (like nausea and hair loss) arise from the fact that chemo kills not only cancer cells but also any other cells that happen to be dividing rapidly at the time, such as hair follicles or cells lining the gut.

If you could slow down the growth of normal cells by fasting, that would help protect your healthy cells from the chemo while leaving the cancer cells vulnerable to attack. But could you imagine doing a fast while going through chemo? And would it be safe?

Nora Quinn

A few years ago I met Nora Quinn, a former judge who, like Jenni Russell, had decided to give periodic fasting a go.

Nora had invasive breast cancer and she had already been through several courses of chemotherapy and radiation, which had made her feel terrible.

When she read about Valter's work she decided to do a seven-day, water-only fast, before, during, and after her next course of chemotherapy. It was tough. But Nora felt it was worth it because she had far fewer side effects from the chemo and made a much more rapid recovery.

More recently, she had a scare when routine mammography revealed what looked like a cyst, or possibly a new cancer, in her untreated breast. While waiting for further tests, she did a seven-day water fast ". . . and it disappeared. All gone. Still gone."

"I am so pleased that doctors are now taking fasting seriously," she told me. "But medicine is so slow to change. Which is frustrating."

The Fast Mimicking Diet

While he is delighted that periodic fasting worked so well for Nora, Valter knows that there are not many cancer patients who are prepared to do a water-only fast—or for whom it is suitable. So, with funding from the National Cancer Institute and other organizations, Valter and his team have created what he now calls a "Fast Mimicking Diet" (FMD). This is not a full-on fast, but a five-day diet where you live on about 800 calories a day. It is a moderately low-protein diet made up of a carefully balanced mix of vegetables, olive oil, and nuts.

If you want to find out more about the FMD, then I recommend you get Valter's recent book, *The Longevity Diet*, where he goes into the pros and cons in depth. You can also get more information from his website, www.valterlongo.com.

The FMD is currently the subject of at least a dozen different clinical trials being carried out in medical centers in Italy, the Netherlands, Germany, and the US. One is a trial of 250 women with breast cancer, half of whom will be randomized to FMD, to see if it really does improve tolerance and survival after chemo compared to standard treatment. Results from some of these trials are expected in late 2019.

2. THE 5:2 APPROACH

Periodic fasting could be a great way to reset your immune system if you have a problem like Jenni Russell, and may turn out to be really helpful for people undergoing chemotherapy, but I was looking for something different: an easy way to lose weight and reverse my diabetes.

So back in 2012, after talking to lots of other scientists, I came up with my own form of intermittent fasting which I thought would be safe and more doable. I called it the "5:2 diet." I decided that for five days a week I would eat healthily and, on my two fasting days, I would cut down to roughly 25% of my normal intake, which would mean I would be eating around 600 calories a day.

I didn't think it would make any difference which days I fasted, so I opted for Tuesdays and Thursdays. This was mainly a process of elimination. I didn't want to do Fridays or the weekends, for obvious social reasons. Fasting on a Monday also struck me as an unappealing way to start the week. I tried doing my fasts back to back (Tuesdays and Wednesdays), but I found that inconvenient.

Given the slightly haphazard way in which I came up with the 5:2 regimen, I was amazed and delighted by how popular and effective it has proved to be, not just for me but for so many other people too. People like Denise.

Denise, who is 51, realized she had to do something when, a few years ago, she noticed that she was short of breath just walking up the stairs. She went to her doctor and was told that she was borderline diabetic. That really worried her, as her mom has type 2 diabetes.

"I saw your book and I followed it to the letter. I lost 35.2 lb in the first eight weeks and I've lost another 13.2 lb since then. I am not borderline diabetic anymore, in fact I'm healthier than I have ever been. I saw my doctor yesterday and he said I am a model patient."

Once she started to lose weight, she adopted other healthy habits. This is often what happens. From being caught up in a vicious cycle of anxiety and comfort eating, you switch over to a virtuous cycle where you feel so much better that you want to make changes to your life. As Denise told me, "My sleep improved. I felt more energetic. I began doing mindfulness. I joined a walking group. The walking group got me into swimming."

So what kept her on track? "Knowing that I've kept the weight off and knowing that it can go back on unless I'm careful. My husband is one of those people who is tall and thin and can eat lots of pizza. I know I can't. I've accepted that. It's accepting, in your head, that you can live your life differently that is so important."

Were there tricky moments? "Lots. I remember vividly one evening when I was wandering round the house looking for a box of chocolates that was left over from Christmas. Fortunately, it was well hidden so eventually I gave up and read a book instead . . . My husband and kids are very supportive. They can see what a big difference it has made to my health and my confidence."

New studies

Terrific as it is to receive feedback from successful dieters like Denise, ultimately a diet program has to be backed up by scientific studies. So what studies have been done and what do they show?

The 5:2 and raised blood sugar

In July 2018 an Australian group, based at the Sansom Institute of Health Research, published the results of a long-term study testing the effects of the 5:2 on people with raised blood sugar levels.[10]

To give you some idea of just how long these sorts of studies take: the Australians started planning this one in 2014, completed it by the end of 2017, and published the results in July 2018.

For the study, 137 overweight or obese people with raised blood sugar levels were randomly allocated to either the 5:2 approach or a standard weight-loss diet for a year. After being carefully weighed and measured, both groups were given information booklets about their respective diets, with sample menus, and sent away to get on with it.

What's so great about this particular study is that the volunteers weren't given special foods or meal replacements or lots of professional support, as commonly happens in diet studies. They just got advice and, for the first few months, were offered regular meetings with a trained dietician.

The point was to try and replicate real-world experience, rather than something that could only be done with lots of expensive professional help.

So, what happened? For the first three months of the study both groups were really good at sticking to their diets, with 97% of the 5:2ers staying on track, compared to 90% of those on a standard diet.

By the end of the year about a third of the volunteers had stopped doing their allocated diet, either because they had hit their goals or because they were tired of dieting. The drop-out rate was higher among the standard dieters than the 5:2ers. In fact, the 5:2ers found that, if they did stop the diet, for whatever reason, it was easy to pick it up again—whereas the people doing the standard diet tended to give up for good.

And weight loss? The people who had been allocated to the 5:2 diet had lost, and kept off, an average of 15.6 lb. Which was 4.6 lb more than the standard dieters. They also lost more fat and saw significant improvements in their blood sugar levels.

Some did better than others. The top 20% in the 5:2ers group managed to lose and keep off an average of 27.5 lb, which was 8.8 lb more than the top 20% in the standard dieting group.

The researchers concluded that the 5:2 diet is safe

and effective, even in people with type 2 diabetes, as long as it is well monitored.

The 5:2 and breast cancer

In 2013, soon after *The FastDiet* was published, Dr. Michelle Harvie and Professor Tony Howell from Manchester University published the results of a study looking at the effects of two days of calorie restriction on 115 middle-aged women.[11]

The women were divided into three groups. One group was asked to stick to a 1,500-calorie Mediterranean diet, while a second group (called "two day dieters") was asked to go on a Mediterranean diet five days a week, but to eat a 650-calorie, low-carbohydrate version on the other two days. A third group was asked to avoid carbohydrates for two days a week, but was otherwise not calorie-restricted.

After three months, the two-day dieters had lost an average of 13 lb, almost twice as much as the daily dieters, and they had also lost far more belly fat. Unlike the regular dieters, the two-day dieters saw a significant improvement in their insulin resistance. Those who stuck with the two-day diet for more than three months lost an average of 13.2 lb; some lost over 30.8 lb. So, another hugely encouraging study for anyone who wants to give 5:2 a go.

In another more recent study,[12] Dr. Harvie asked 23 overweight, premenopausal women at high risk of breast cancer to cut back their calories, two days a week, for one menstrual cycle. As well as standard tests they agreed to have breast biopsies.

Over the course of a month, the women not only lost an average of 6.6 lb, most of it body fat, but in most of the women there were significant changes in the activity of genes associated with breast cancer.

The first human trial on the impact of the 5:2 on the brain

Another reason why I am so enthusiastic about spreading the intermittent-fasting message is its potential impact on preventing dementia. Dementia is now the leading cause of death in the UK. Worldwide, there are more than 50 million people with it, and this number is expected to triple by 2050.

New approaches are desperately needed because the tragedy of dementia is that once you have symptoms nothing can stop it. Despite billions spent on research, drugs are largely ineffective.

And that's where Mark Mattson, professor of neuroscience at the National Institute on Aging, comes in. He has spent decades researching the impact of intermittent fasting on the brain, showing how it can help combat diseases like dementia, Parkinson's, and memory loss.

Much of Mark's work in the past has been with animals, trying to understand exactly why intermittent fasting is so good for brain health. A few years ago, he showed me an experiment he was doing with mice that had been specially bred to develop Alzheimer's. These mice normally develop Alzheimer's when they are about 12 months old, the equivalent to being a middle-aged human. The mice he put on an intermittent-fasting diet didn't develop dementia until they were well into old age.

When they died, he examined their brains and he found that those put on an intermittent-fasting diet had grown new brain cells, particularly in the hippocampus area, which is essential for learning and memory

Why does this happen? Well, Mark's team has recently shown the importance of ketones in this process. Ketones, as I mentioned earlier, are produced by your liver when you "flip the metabolic switch," and your body goes from burning sugar to burning fat for fuel. Despite what some "health experts" claim, your brain will run perfectly well on ketones. In fact, in many ways it seems to prefer ketones as a fuel source.

As the Greeks discovered, more than 2,000 years ago, making people fast and go into a ketotic state is an effective way to treat and prevent epilepsy. The first low-carb, ketogenic diet was developed in the 1930s as a treatment for epilepsy in children and is still used today.

So why are ketones so good for the brain? "Because ketones act directly on nerve cells to stimulate production of a protein called BDNF," Mark told me.

BDNF, Brain Derived Neurotrophic Factor, is a protein that in turn stimulates the creation of new brain cells and new brain cell connections. BDNF is also a natural antidepressant, which might explain why so many people find the 5:2 surprisingly easy to stick to.

Mark's animal research showing that intermittent fasting can improve memory and delay dementia is fascinating. But, for me, the really exciting news is that he is just coming to the end of the first human trial to see if the 5:2 diet can protect and boost the *human* brain.

For this study, he recruited 40 people (between the ages of 55 and 70), all with proven insulin resistance, which puts them at increased risk of developing dementia and other memory problems. The volunteers were then randomly allocated to either a 5:2 diet, or a control group, who were offered "healthy living" counseling instead.

At the start of the study the volunteers underwent extensive tests, which included measuring their weight, insulin resistance, and the level of ketones in their blood. They also did lots of cognitive tests (to assess memory and how on the ball they were, mentally), and had brain scans and lumbar punctures (a procedure in which a needle is inserted into the spinal cord to measure biomarkers for Alzheimer's).

The volunteers had to go back to the clinic for repeat tests every two weeks until the end of the experiment, which ran for 12 weeks.

So what happened?

Frustratingly, I can't tell you because the study is not yet complete. When I asked Mark, all he could say was that "the interim data is encouraging." He's expecting to publish the results some time in 2019. If you sign up for our newsletter at thefast800.com, I will let you know what happens.

In the meantime, if you are considering intermittent fasting as a way of delaying the onset of dementia, Mark says you should get going sooner rather than later.

The changes which lead to dementia occur very early, probably decades before you start to have learning and memory problems. That's why it's critical to start dietary regimens early on, when you are young or middle-aged, so that you can slow down the development of these damaging processes in the brain and live to be 90 with your brain functioning perfectly well.

As he points out, there are a lot of pressures not to change. "The food industry is not going to make money if people start skipping meals," he told me. "Nor is the pharmaceutical industry. Our challenge is to communicate the science so that people understand what they can do and then take action."

Like Mark, I'm convinced that our brains benefit from short fasts, which is why I still do them. But I'm also convinced that intermittent fasting has other measurable health benefits, including its effects on the heart. So that's where we'll turn to next.

The 5:2 and the heart

"Have a heart that never hardens," said Charles Dickens. Although he didn't mean it in a medical sense, it is excellent advice. After dementia, heart disease is the next biggest killer in the UK. Even if you survive a heart attack, it can leave a devastating legacy.

Despite it being a universal symbol of love, the heart is actually just an extraordinarily good pump. No bigger than a fist, it pushes 5 liters of blood through the 59,962 miles of blood vessels in your body 70 times a minute. That's 100,000 times a day and, if you keep it in good shape, it should go on doing so about three billion times during your lifetime.

The trouble is, many of us have hearts that are aging faster than they should, which could be why they are often the first bit of the human machine to go seriously wrong. If you'd like to find out how "old" your heart really is, then go to the NHS website and fill in the questionnaire (www.nhs.uk/conditions/nhs-health-check /check-your-heart-age-tool).

So how can you keep your heart young? By eating a Mediterranean-style diet (see Chapter 4), keeping active (see Chapter 5), and reducing stress (see Chapter 6), you will take years off your heart age and cut your risk of having a heart attack or stroke.

Going on the 5:2 will also improve your heart health, by helping you lose weight and lower your blood sugar levels. In a recent study,[13] 27 overweight men and women were randomly put on either a 5:2 diet or a standard diet and asked to lose 5% of their body weight. Those allocated to the 5:2 diet managed to do it in 59 days, while those on the standard diet took 73 days.

There was a much bigger fall in blood pressure among the 5:2ers (down by 9% compared to 3%) and the researchers also found that when they gave the dieters a fatty meal the 5:2ers were able to clear the fat from their blood much faster. So it was another very encouraging 5:2 result.

As you'll see on page 127, getting your blood pressure and blood sugar levels measured are some of the tests I recommend you have done before starting the Fast800. That way, you can see what shape your heart is in and if the answer is "not great," it will give you even more incentive to stick to the diet. Acting before you have a heart attack is far, far better than waiting and hoping.

3. TIME RESTRICTED EATING

The final form of intermittent fasting I want to tell you about is called Time Restricted Eating (TRE). It has recently become popular, particularly among millennials, body builders, and celebrities. The actor Hugh Jackman says his Wolverine physique was made possible by doing a form of TRE called 16:8. When I have my hair cut, I like to chat to the person trimming my locks. These days they all seem to be doing TRE.

The rules of TRE are very simple: you try to eat most of your calories within a narrow time window, such as 12 hours (also known as 12:12). Once you have decided on your time window (perhaps 9 a.m. to 9 p.m.), you don't eat or drink anything that contains calories outside that period.

You can start doing TRE by simply having your evening meal a bit earlier and your breakfast a bit later (12:12). That way you extend your normal overnight fast (the time when you are asleep and not eating) by a few hours. Once you have gotten used to this you can move to the 14:10 or even, like Hugh Jackman, to the 16:8 (where you eat all your calories in an eight-hour window, such as between midday and 8 p.m., and fast for 16 hours).

How does TRE work?

The idea of "time-restricted eating" is not new; more than 2,500 years ago Buddha told his followers that, if they made it their practice to stop eating after their midday meal and fast until the following morning, they would achieve enhanced mental clarity and a sense of well-being. But the person who really put the science into TRE is Dr. Satchin Panda, a professor at the Salk Institute in San Diego, one of the world's leading research centers for biomedicine and life sciences.

I first came across his work in 2012 when I was researching intermittent fasting for *The FastDiet*. As I was trawling the internet, I found a study that he and his colleagues had just published called "Time-restricted feeding without reducing caloric intake prevents metabolic diseases in mice fed a high-fat diet."[14] It blew me away.

For this study they took two groups of genetically identical mice and fed them a high-fat, high-sugar diet. All the mice got exactly the same amount of food to eat, the only difference being that the mice in one group were allowed to eat whenever they wanted, while the mice in the other group had to eat their food within an eight-hour time window. This meant that there were 16 hours of the day in which they were, involuntarily, fasting.

After 100 days there were some remarkable differences between the two groups. The mice who had no time restrictions on eating their sugary fatty feast had, as expected, put on huge amounts of weight, particularly in visceral fat. As a result they had developed high cholesterol and high blood sugars, and were already showing signs of liver damage.

What was astonishing was that the genetically

identical mice, who had been eating the same food, except in an eight-hour window, were protected from these changes. They put on far less weight and suffered much less liver damage.

TRE trials with humans

After reading Dr. Panda's study I was keen to see if TRE works just as well with people. So I was delighted when in 2017, I was asked to get involved in one of the first randomized human trials of TRE. The study was designed and carried out by Dr. Jonathan Johnston at the University of Surrey.[15]

For the study, he recruited 16 healthy volunteers. After they'd had their body fat, blood sugar levels, blood fats (triglycerides), and cholesterol levels measured, they were randomly assigned to one of two groups, the blues or the reds.

The blues, who were the control group, were asked to carry on as normal. The reds were asked to stick to their normal diet but eat their breakfast 90 minutes later, and their dinner 90 minutes earlier. This meant that for an extra three hours each day they were going without food (fasting). The experiment ran for 10 weeks and everyone kept a food and sleep diary to ensure that they were eating the same amount as normal.

At the end of the 10 weeks, we gathered all the

volunteers together and repeated the tests. The group who had eaten breakfast later and dinner earlier had lost more body fat, an average of around 3.5 lb. They also saw bigger falls in blood sugar levels and cholesterol than the control group. The differences weren't huge but they were significant and most of the volunteers said they had found it relatively easy to do.

In another small study,[16] Dr. Panda teamed up with Dr. Krista Varady of the University of Chicago. They recruited 23 obese men and women and asked them to eat only between 10 a.m. and 6 p.m. They were allowed to eat and drink whatever they wanted within those hours. Outside those hours they were allowed nothing but water, black tea, black coffee, or diet soda.

The subjects stuck to it (mostly) and lost an average 4.4 lb of fat over the next 12 weeks. Again, not a huge weight loss, but there was a big fall in their insulin resistance and they also reported sleeping better, having less hunger at bedtime, and feeling more energetic.

I've given TRE a go (see page 66) and I do think it is worth trying. I think it is particularly helpful when you are confining yourself to 800 calories a day, which is why I have included it as part of my program.

The optimum fasting window

The research done on animals suggests that fasting for at least 16 hours ensures the greatest benefit, but for many people that may be impractical. So what is the least you can get away with?

Dr. Panda says, "Most of your body fat burning happens six to eight hours after finishing your last meal and increases almost exponentially after a full 12 hours, which means that going longer than 12 hours is likely to be particularly beneficial. Once you've achieved your desired weight loss you can go back to an 11- or 12-hour window and maintain body weight."

He recommends that you don't jump straight into doing something like 16:8 (fasting for 16 hours and eating for 8), but instead ease into it. Start with trying to eat within a 12-hour window, then after a couple of weeks reduce it to 10 hours, and if you are still feeling good, cut down to eight hours. It's a bit like exercise. It wouldn't be a good idea to try running a marathon without at least a bit of training.

And does it matter when you do your fasting/ eating?

Although many of us like to unwind with a big meal at the end of the day, it is better to eat most of your calories earlier, if you can. That's because your body is much better at handling sugar and fat in the morning or afternoon, rather than in the evening. By evening your body is getting ready to close down for the night and will not appreciate being forced to restart the complex process of digestion.

To test this claim, I decided to do a little experiment on myself. After an overnight fast (12 hours without anything to eat or drink) I had some blood taken by a friendly doctor. Then, at precisely 10 a.m., I had a classic British fry-up, with lots of bacon, eggs, and sausage.

Straight after the meal I had more blood taken, and then again every half hour for the next few hours. After that, I had nothing but water until the late evening.

Twelve hours after eating breakfast, at 10 p.m., I had my second meal of the day. It was exactly the same as I had had for breakfast. Bacon, eggs, and sausage. Again, my blood was taken regularly over the next few hours before I eventually decided I had had enough and crawled into bed.

When the results of the blood tests came back they were pretty shocking. They showed that after eating a full English fry-up in the morning my blood sugar levels rose quickly, but returned to normal within a couple of hours. The levels of fat in my blood also rose fast, then began to drop after about three hours.

What happened in the evening, however, was very different. Despite eating exactly the same meal, my blood sugar levels went up and stayed high for several hours. The fat levels in my blood were even worse, still rising at two in the morning, four hours after I had finished eating. I don't know when they stopped rising because after that I went to bed.

What is clear from many studies is that our bodies don't like having to deal with lots of food late at night. A midnight snack will have a much worse impact on you than the same food eaten earlier in the day.

TRE and acid reflux

If you suffer from acid reflux (heartburn) I would strongly recommend finishing eating well before bedtime. If you eat within three hours of going to bed, there is a risk that partially digested, acid-drenched food will start coming back up your esophagus. Trying to ease heartburn by having a milky drink, or a bowl of cereal last thing at night, as many do, will make this worse.

TRE and cancer

As we've seen, going on a 5:2 diet reduces insulin levels, which are an important driver of cancer. Can TRE also help reduce cancer risk?

No one has yet carried out a trial, but researchers did make use of a big study designed for a completely different purpose to find out.

The Women's Healthy Eating and Living (WHEL) trial[17] was hugely expensive. Some 2,400 American women with breast cancer were randomly allocated to either a low-fat diet or given a pamphlet on the benefits of "5 a day." They were then followed for over seven years to see if going low-fat made any difference.

The answer was a resounding "no." Despite reducing their fat intake by 19%, the low-fat dieters were no better off than the control group.

But the great thing about this study, from the point of view of researchers investigating TRE, is that the women were asked to keep detailed records of not only *what* they ate but *when* they ate.

The women whose diaries showed that they had fasted for more than 13 hours a night had 36% less chance of a breast cancer recurrence than those who had been fasting for less than 13 hours. The researchers also found that women who typically ate after 8 p.m. were significantly fatter. Another good reason to skip the late-night snack.

TRE as part of the Fast800

TRE works extremely well with other diets and that's why I recommend giving it a go as part of my new Fast800 program. In many ways it makes intermittent fasting easier (after a relatively brief adjustment period you don't feel hungry and therefore tempted to cheat late at night) and it can be an effective tool for keeping the weight off.

Meri is a great example of what can be achieved. She's 46 years old, slim, youthful, the mother of five children. Yet a couple of years ago she was over 220 lb. Her weight problems started with the birth of her first child.

"I put on nearly 66 lb with my first pregnancy," she told me, "and then I realized I had no idea how to get it off. I did every sort of diet, from Weight Watchers to Jenny Craig, but the weight kept coming back. I was up and down, up and down for 22 years."

Eventually Meri decided she really had to do something about it. So she went on a rapid weight-loss diet.

"I knew if I could see results quickly I would stick with it, and that's been supported by a lot of the stuff I have read. It was difficult at times, making food for the rest of the family and not eating it myself. But I wasn't really distracted by food. In fact, the more that I could see the success, the more motivated I was and the easier it became. I became surprisingly euphoric."

She lost 66 lb in four months. "I didn't really have a goal. The weight kept falling off so I just kept on going. I think you have to readjust your eyeballs at first. You become so much slimmer than you thought was possible. I'm the same size now as I was when I was 20."

Two years after losing all that weight she remains slim and healthy. I asked her how she does it. "I eat mainly vegetables, but I'm not rigid. I'm a vegetarian who sometimes eats meat and a teetotaler who drinks alcohol. I do try to stay away from sugar because I'm a terrible sugar addict."

She has one rule she sticks by. "I try to eat within an eight-hour period each day, so I don't eat after 4 o'clock in the afternoon. Everyone in my family is used to that now. I still sit with them for dinner, I just don't eat. My family realizes that what I've done for my health and therefore for them is so much more important than breaking that rule."

In summary:

- There are different ways to do intermittent fasting.
- A five-day fast can help reset your immune system and may also enhance the effects of chemotherapy.
- Intermittent fasting activates a process called "autophagy," which literally means "self-eat," and puts your body into repair mode.

- Studies show that the 5:2 is not only good for weight loss and improving your insulin sensitivity, but may also help boost your brain, reduce your risk of heart disease, and lower your blood sugars.
- TRE complements intermittent fasting and can be an effective tool to help you lose weight and keep it off.

3

THE CASE FOR RAPID WEIGHT LOSS

One of the other major revolutions in the weight-loss world, alongside intermittent fasting, has been the return of very rapid weight-loss diets. Diets in which you reduce your intake to 800 calories each day, every day, for up to 20 weeks. Diets on which you can expect to lose around 30.8 lb in three months.

We've been repeatedly told that rapid weight loss is ineffective and futile: that if you lose weight fast you will put it back on even faster. But this is not borne out by the latest research. Here are a few things that I learned from weight-loss experts in the course of researching this book:

1. Rapid weight loss is no more likely to lead to rapid weight regain than slow and steady dieting.
2. People who lose weight fast are more likely to hit their targets than those who do it slowly.

3. The amount of weight you lose in the first few weeks of a diet predicts how much you will lose and keep off in the long run.

I'm going to show you how you can safely and effectively incorporate very rapid weight loss into my Fast800 program. But first, let's look at three new research studies, showing how successful and effective a rapid weight-loss diet can be.

The DIRECT study

As I mentioned in the introduction to this book, in early 2014 I came across what seemed like a crazy claim: that people who follow a rapid weight-loss diet not only lose a lot of weight, fast, but by doing so also clean fat out of their livers and reverse their type 2 diabetes.

This audacious claim was being made by Dr. Roy Taylor, professor of Medicine and Metabolism at Newcastle University and one of Europe's leading diabetes experts. When we first met he showed me some of the studies he'd done showing that type 2 diabetes (the sort of diabetes you get when you are older) can be put into remission, perhaps even "cured," by a rapid weight-loss diet.

As he explained, the reason most people get type 2 diabetes is that they have too much fat around the tummy. Unlike the fat on your bottom or thighs, the fat on your tummy, visceral fat, infiltrates your liver and pancreas, and stops them "talking to each other." This can, in time, lead to type 2 diabetes.

Just because your pancreas has gone quiet, however, doesn't mean it can't be revived. And the best way to do that? Lose a lot of weight. Fast.

Roy told me that I'd managed to get my blood sugars back to normal by doing the 5:2 because I had lost over 10% of my body weight, draining fat from my liver and pancreas.

The implications of what Roy was saying were huge. Type 2 diabetes is the fastest-growing chronic disease, worldwide. There are more than 400 million people with the condition and though drugs help control symptoms, they have limited impact on the underlying disease.

If Roy was right and people with type 2 diabetes really can restore their blood sugars to normal without drugs, then this was a massive breakthrough. But, though Roy had done human trials showing it could be done safely through diet, most doctors remained skeptical.

"They don't believe patients will do it," he told me, "and they don't believe it will work."

Roy knew he needed to run a really big trial to convince the skeptics. Together with a friend and colleague, Professor Mike Lean of Glasgow University, Roy persuaded the charity Diabetes UK to donate £1.6m to run a study that they called DIRECT (DIabetes REmission Clinical Trial).[18]

Roy and Mike started by recruiting 298 patients from GP practices in Scotland and the northeast. The patients were then randomly allocated to either an 800-calorie-a-day diet, made up largely of meal replacement shakes, with behavioral support, or to following the best conventional advice and support. The patients were then followed for at least a year. The whole study took more than four years.

When the results were published in *The Lancet*, in February 2018, they were astonishing:

- Those on the 800-calorie diet had lost an average of 22 lb, compared to 2.2 lb in the control group.
- A quarter of those on the 800-calorie diet had lost more than 33 lb. None of those in the control group managed this.
- Nearly half of the 800-calorie group managed to bring their blood sugars back down to normal, despite coming off all their diabetes drugs. The more weight they lost, the higher their chance of bringing their pancreas back to life: 86% of those who lost more than 33 lb went into remission (i.e., their blood sugars returned to normal despite the fact they had come off all medication).

Mike was delighted with the findings and told me, "Given our results, it should be considered unethical *not* to give people with type 2 diabetes access to the necessary support for at least a good try at a remission. Most patients want to try, and it would save the NHS a lot of money."

Roy was also thrilled by just how clear their findings were. He thinks this study will really change the treatment of diabetes but acknowledges that there are still important questions that need to be answered. The scientists will continue to track patients to see how many keep the weight off and diabetes at bay.

Mike's story

As I have explained, soon after I met Roy, I wrote, with his support, *The 8-Week Blood Sugar Diet*, outlining a similar regimen of 800 calories a day for rapid weight loss. Since then I have heard from thousands of people who have followed the diet and reversed their diabetes.

People like Mike Cunningham, who'd had type 2 diabetes for many years before reading my book and deciding to try an 800-calorie approach. He was motivated to change by what happened to his younger sister, Angela.

"My beautiful sister Angela," he wrote, "first developed diabetes when she was pregnant."

Nearly one in ten women develops gestational diabetes—high blood sugar levels—when they are pregnant. Most find that their blood sugars return to normal after they have given birth. Angela's didn't. Although she was on medication, she later developed one of the common complications of diabetes, an infection in her leg.

The infection turned septic. Despite antibiotics, it got so bad she had to have part of her leg amputated. She spent another 16 weeks in intensive care as her doctors battled to save her life. They failed. She died, aged just 45.

"The memory of Angie and her life support being switched off helped me start on the diet and kept me going," Mike wrote. "I was determined never to give in to diabetes or simply rely on medication."

When he started he was 214 lb. In a couple of months he had got down to 152 lb. As the fat melted away, his waist also shrunk, from an unhealthy 37.5 inches to a very healthy 32.5 inches.

His blood sugar levels fell dramatically, as did his cholesterol. He was able to come off all medication including insulin, metformin, and gliclazide.

"There were hurdles," he said, "such as family celebrations. My work takes me away from home and I find it difficult finding restaurants or hotels with healthy options."

But with time it got easier, because he and his partner discovered the pleasures of eating real food.

"I want to thank everyone involved in this work from the bottom of my heart. I have learned so much about good foods and I have a much greater awareness of which foods are good for me personally. I now avoid processed foods totally. My life has been transformed."

The PREVIEW study

Going on an 800-calorie rapid weight-loss diet is challenging, but people with type 2 diabetes have a lot of motivation to do it. So would the rapid weight-loss approach work for people who don't have type 2 diabetes? Would they stick to it?

Two other big studies, which published results in 2018, suggest that it would.

The PREVIEW study[19] was set up to prevent people with prediabetes from developing diabetes. Prediabetes, where you have raised blood sugars, not yet in the diabetic range, is incredibly common. Around a third of the adult population have it, but unless you've been tested you won't know because there are usually no symptoms.

When the study started, the volunteers—2,326 middle-aged men and women from eight countries (Britain, Denmark, Finland, Holland, Bulgaria, Spain, New Zealand, and Australia)—all had prediabetes. Once they'd had the usual tests done, they were asked to go on an 800-calorie diet for eight weeks.

Results of this massive study, published in August 2018, show that they lost an average of 24 lb in just eight weeks. Most of this was fat, with their waists shrinking by an average of 4 inches.

Many of the participants managed to get their blood sugar levels back to normal and there were few side effects, apart from constipation (7%) and headaches (3%). The best way to counter both of these is to drink more water.

The plan is to follow these people for many more years to see if they manage to keep weight off and diabetes at bay.

The DROPLET trial

Hot on the heels of DIRECT and PREVIEW came another 800-calorie a day rapid weight-loss trial, this time carried out by researchers at Oxford University. For this trial, called DROPLET,[20] 278 obese adults were either assigned to a regimen where they got 800 calories a day in the form of meal replacement soups and shakes, or put on a standard slow and steady diet program.

Those on the meal replacement regimen were asked to stick to it for eight weeks, before gradually switching to eating real food. They also got behavioral support throughout.

At the end of a year the group on the rapid weight-loss diet had lost an average of 23.5 lb, while those in the standard dieting group had lost 6.6 lb.

Susan Jebb, professor of diet and population health at Oxford University and the lead researcher, was delighted by the results. "It's phenomenal—extraordinary—like nothing we've seen in primary care before."

She thinks one of the reasons that the rapid weight-loss group did so well is because rapid weight loss is very motivating: "The excitement gets them through the first few difficult weeks . . . We need to capitalize on all that enthusiasm that people have at the beginning to really lose weight and get off as much weight as they possibly can."

Like other weight-loss specialists I spoke to, she said that science did not support the often-repeated claims that people's metabolic rates will crash, never to recover, or that people who lose weight fast put it on even faster. Instead she said studies consistently show that early weight loss predicts long-term weight loss.

"Weight loss at four weeks, certainly at 12 weeks, is a really good predictor of what will happen later. In a previous study we showed that weight loss at 12 weeks predicted weight loss at two years."

Above all, Professor Jebb is frustrated by how slowly things are changing. "This is an area of medicine where our understanding has come on in leaps and bounds but practice has not changed. If we had a new drug which had achieved what DIRECT (Roy Taylor's diabetes study) had achieved it would be screamed from the roof tops . . . We have something which is effective and which is really cheap. And we are not doing it. I find that unbelievable."

Q&A

If I do a rapid weight-loss diet, won't I put the weight straight back on?

Not according to the experts I've spoken to. The studies I've just quoted ran for over a year and weight regain was no more a problem for those who lost weight rapidly than those who lost it gradually. In fact, rapid weight-loss dieters lost and kept off far more weight.

As Professor Mike Lean, head of nutrition at Glasgow University, told me, "Losing weight slowly is torture. The people who do it rapidly see better results in the long run. Contrary to the belief of dieticians, people who lose weight more quickly, more emphatically, are more likely to keep it off in the long term."

It's a view that Susie, a GP, would agree with. She lost 34 lb in just eight weeks using my Blood Sugar Diet approach and has kept it off for more than three years. "I feel full of energy. Happier. I feel in control of my hunger for the first time."

An Australian study which involved 200 obese volunteers being put on an 800-calorie rapid weight-loss diet for 12 weeks found that not only did they lose more weight than steady dieters, but four years later they were still leaner.[21] As two leading weight-loss experts, Dr. Corby Martin and Professor Kishore Gadde from Pennington Biomedical Research Center, Baton Rouge, put it, "The myth that rapid weight loss is associated with rapid weight gain is no more true than Aesop's fables."

That said, it is important that if you go on a rapid weight-loss diet you do it properly. If you are on medication, you must talk to your doctor before starting.

Whatever diet you decide to follow, it is vital that you are getting enough daily protein (at least 50–60g a day), otherwise you will lose muscle. You also need to be sure you are getting enough of all the other essential nutrients—you should avoid going on one of those crazy cabbage soup or green juice diets, for example. The menus in this book were created to be safe and sustainable.

Won't my metabolism crash if I go on a rapid weight-loss diet?

Fear of going into "starvation mode" is one of the reasons so many people think diets, particularly rapid weight-loss diets, don't work.

This belief is based on the Minnesota Starvation Experiment,[22] a study carried out during World War Two in which slim young volunteers lived on a low-calorie diet (around 1,500 calories a day) made up largely of turnips and potatoes.

After six months on this very low-protein diet, when their body fat had fallen to less than 10%, their metabolic rate (the energy the body uses to keep itself going) crashed. This was an extreme situation.

A more recent experiment on the effects of short-term calorie restriction,[23] produced very different results. In this experiment 11 healthy volunteers were asked to fast for 84 hours (just under four days).

The researchers found that the volunteers' metabolic rate went up while they were fasting. By Day 3 it had risen, on average, by 14%.

Whichever way you lose weight, fast or slow, your metabolism will slow down simply because you are now carrying less weight around. That's why it is so important, as you lose weight, to remain active. What you eat as you lose weight is also critically important (see below).

But what about the longer term?

One of the best ways to preserve your muscle and your metabolic rate is to not only stick to 800 calories but go low-carb for the initial stage of the diet. In a recent Spanish study,[24] 20 obese people were put on an 800-calorie very low-carb diet. The participants lost an average of 44 lb in four months (of which 80% was fat) but their metabolic rate only dropped by 8%.

The researchers said this was because the combination of low-carb and low-calorie put them into a state of mild ketosis, which not only helped to preserve muscle but also meant they were less hungry.

The Fast800 is a mildly ketogenic diet, where you are eating a much higher ratio of fat and protein to carbs than you normally would, especially during the rapid weight-loss phase. More on that later.

If I do put the weight back on, will I be worse off than I was before?

Nobody who goes on a diet intends to put the weight back on, but it happens. When I asked Professor Jebb if that mattered she said, emphatically, no. "The harmful effects of obesity come from how big you are and from how long you've carried that extra weight. Even if you have a few years where you are lighter than you would have been, that brings very substantial health benefits."

She says that you should weigh yourself regularly and, if you find you are putting weight back on, you should act as quickly as possible to stop it progressing. A few pounds can soon turn into a lot of pounds.

What about exercising on a rapid weight-loss diet?

There is no reason to stop exercising because it will, if anything, help put you into ketosis faster and preserve muscle mass. That said, I wouldn't recommend trying something that requires burning a lot of calories, such as running a marathon. I find that doing push-ups and going for runs is both possible and usefully distracting when I am fasting. In fact, I find that my right knee, which has a touch of osteoarthritis (thanks to an old sports injury) gets much better when I am fasting. Which makes the running easier.

Who shouldn't embark on a rapid weight-loss diet?

As with any weight-loss diet, if you have any reason for concern you should always check with your doctor first. Because the Fast800 is a powerful therapeutic tool, it is important that you check whether any of the following apply to you before starting.

Don't do the diet if you:

- Are under 18 years of age.
- Are breastfeeding, pregnant, or undergoing fertility treatment. However, if you are pregnant and there is a risk of (or previous history of) gestational diabetes, you might consider the Med-style diet.
- Are underweight and/or have a history or suspicion of an eating disorder.
- Have a significant psychiatric disorder or a history of substance abuse.
- Are under active medical investigation or treatment, or have a significant medical condition affecting your ability to comply with a diet.
- Have had a recent cardiac event, myocardial infarction, or cerebrovascular accident (less than three months ago) or other heart abnormalities.

- Have uncontrolled heart disease, uncontrolled hypertension, or kidney failure.
- Are unwell, have a fever, are frail, or recovering from significant surgery (less than six months ago).

Cautions—discuss with your doctor if any of the following apply:

- You have a significant underlying medical condition.
- You are on insulin—you will need a detailed assessment and education by a health professional to plan a suitable reduction in medication/insulin to avoid a potentially dangerous drop in blood sugar (hypo).
- You have type 2 diabetes and are on medication. Your medication may need to be reduced or stopped as blood sugars improve and to avoid hypos.
- You are on certain diabetic medication and have "hypoglycemia unawareness."
- You are on blood pressure medication. This may need to be reduced or stopped as blood pressure improves.
- You are taking other medications, e.g., warfarin.
- You have moderate or severe retinopathy; you will need extra screening within six months as

retinopathy can sometimes get worse when blood sugar improves.

- You have epilepsy (though there is some evidence that a low-carb keto diet can improve epilepsy).
- You are pregnant: clearly avoiding fasting/low-calorie diets is wise.

If you have type 2 diabetes or prediabetes do visit the DIRECT study website for more information and dietary advice.[25]

You should also be cautious if you have a history of gallstone problems. In Professor Taylor's study, one person did complain of cholecystitis (inflammation of the gallbladder) after being on the diet, though it is not certain that the diet was responsible. Gallstone formation is also associated with having diabetes and being overweight.

Rapid weight loss is challenging (which is also part of its benefit). So, if you are not suited to fasting, you may prefer simply to follow the Med-style, low-carb recipes in this book without significantly reducing calories.

4

WHY I LOVE THE MEDITERRANEAN DIET

The recipes in this book are based on a Mediterranean-style diet, a way of eating that is rich in healthy natural fats, nuts, and fish, as well as veggies and legumes, which are packed with disease-fighting vitamins and minerals.

The reason I am such a fan of the Mediterranean diet is not just because it tastes great but because there is so much solid scientific evidence that adopting this lifestyle will cut your risk of heart disease, cancer, type 2 diabetes, depression, and dementia. Even when taken up later in middle age, it has been shown to increase life expectancy.

What can be confusing about the term "Mediterranean diet" is that it is not the sort of food that you would typically associate with your holidays in Italy or Greece. It does not, for instance, include lots of pizza and pasta, or the sort of sticky puddings you might be offered in a Greek restaurant.

The Mediterranean diet I'm writing about is the traditional one of the people who lived around the Mediterranean Sea before they, like so much of the planet, adopted junk food.

In many Mediterranean countries today, vegetables, fish, and olive oil have been displaced by sweets, fizzy drinks, and fast food. In fact, only around 10% of modern Italians eat a traditional Mediterranean diet, with dire consequences for their waists. Italian children, who a generation ago were slim and healthy, are now almost as fat as their American counterparts. Strangely enough, Scandinavians are far more likely to eat a Mediterranean-style diet than the people living in Mediterranean countries.

So, what exactly is a healthy Mediterranean diet?

There are lots of different versions of the Mediterranean diet out there. My approach is based on one of the biggest and most important nutrition studies ever carried out: the PREDIMED study.[26]

In this 2013 study, Spanish researchers recruited over 7,400 overweight, middle-aged Spanish men and women and randomly allocated them to either a Mediterranean or a low-fat diet. Both groups were encouraged to eat lots of fresh fruit, vegetables, and legumes (such as beans, lentils, and peas). They were discouraged from consuming sugary drinks, cakes, sweets, or pastries and from eating too much processed meat such as bacon or salami.

Those allocated to the Mediterranean diet were asked to eat plenty of eggs, nuts, and oily fish and use lots of olive oil, and encouraged to eat some dark chocolate and enjoy the occasional glass of wine with their evening meal.

In contrast, the low-fat diet group were told to eat low-fat dairy products and plenty of starchy foods such as bread, potatoes, pasta, and rice.

The researchers followed the volunteers for years, getting them to fill in food diaries and keeping a check on their health via medical examinations, questionnaires, and blood and urine samples. All volunteers were given an "M score," according to how closely they stuck to the Mediterranean diet.

Within three years, dramatic differences between the two groups appeared. Not only were those who had a high M score slimmer, they were also much healthier, slashing their risk of a multitude of diseases. The benefits included:

- 30% reduced risk of heart attack or stroke
- 58% reduced risk of type 2 diabetes
- 51% reduced risk of breast cancer
- A reduced risk of cognitive decline

How to boost your M score

A simple way to boost your M score is to adhere to the following simple rules:

1. *Reduce sugars and starchy carbs*

Cut right back on sugary starchy foods, such as cakes, sweets, cookies, chips, fruit juices, and soft drinks, as these rapidly turn into sugar in your blood, causing sugar spikes, a surge in insulin, and weight gain. Aim to have them less than twice a week.

You also need to watch out for foods that get rapidly converted to sugars in your blood, such as:

- Potatoes, bread, white rice, and white pasta.
- Most breakfast cereals and "instant oats" (steel-cut or rolled oats are okay).
- Sweet, tropical fruits such as mangoes, pineapples, grapes, melons, and bananas as these are high in sugars (fructose). Instead, opt for berries, apples, or pears. Aim for a maximum of 1–2 pieces of fruit a day, ideally eaten after a meal.
- Processed foods. More than 70% of processed foods contain added sugars. You have to read the labels, though the problem is that there are more than 70 different names for sugars.

2. *Increase your consumption of natural healthy fats*

Many people still believe that eating fat will make them fat and that it will clog up their arteries. I hope I have convinced you this is not true. Enjoy healthy fats in foods such as olive oil, salmon, tuna, full-fat dairy, avocado, nuts, and seeds. These natural fats are good for the waist and the heart, and will keep you feeling full for longer.

3. *Eat decent amounts of protein*

This means eating generous amounts of foods such as oily fish, seafood, chicken, some red meat, eggs, tofu, beans, legumes, dairy, and nuts. If you are a vegetarian or vegan there are alternatives (see page 101). You need at least 50–60g of protein a day, every day. As you get older, you need more. That said, you should restrict your intake of processed meats such as sausages, bacon, and salami, as these are not particularly healthy sources of protein. Most contain high levels of salt, nitrates, and other preservatives.

4. *Eat plenty of green and colored vegetables*

It is especially important to eat plenty of dark-green leafy vegetables such as spinach, broccoli, cabbage, kale, and salads, as well as colored vegetables—these are very low in calories and contain many essential vitamins and nutrients. They also contain lots of fiber, which the "good" microbes in your gut will benefit from.

5. *Swap to whole grains and legumes*

Eat more "complex carbohydrates," which are rich in fiber. This means swapping white pasta and rice for whole grains and legumes such as: lentils, beans, quinoa, wild rice, and buckwheat. Choose multigrain, seeded, or rye bread over white. Again, the good bacteria in your gut will thrive on the fiber in these foods. But during both the rapid weight loss and 5:2 stages of the diet you should keep your intake of whole grains down. That's because you want to go into mild ketosis and eating grains will stop that happening.

6. *Avoid snacking between meals or late-night grazing*

Grazing stops fat burning. If you must, snack on non-starchy vegetables such as broccoli, cucumber, or celery, or a small handful of nuts or a small piece of cheese. Fruit is not a good choice, particularly when you are trying to lose weight.

7. *Drink healthily*

Plenty of black tea, fruit tea, black coffee, and water. As for alcohol, an occasional glass of red wine with a meal is okay on nonfast days. If you are doing an 800-calorie day, it's best to avoid alcohol altogether.

The Mediterranean diet is more than just a diet. It's about developing a set of habits and making permanent changes to your lifestyle. It involves cutting back on processed, ready-made, and fast foods, and instead opting for whole-food meals cooked, where possible, from scratch. And it is about eating food slowly and enjoying it with family and friends. Too often we eat without taking the time to appreciate what is going in our mouths. So don't eat your meal in front of the TV. Make the effort to savor it fully.

The Med diet and the microbiome

Along with the abundance of vitamins and antioxidants, such as those found in extra-virgin olive oil, there is another, crucial reason why this diet is so superhealthy.

As I discovered while researching a previous book, *The Clever Gut Diet*, eating Mediterranean-style foods has a dramatic and positive effect on your gut microbiome—the trillions of microbes that live there, which are so important for your physical and mental well-being.

The "good" bacteria in your gut, like *Bifidobacterium* and *Lactobacillus*, will turn the fiber you get from your Med meals into chemicals called short-chain fatty acids (SCFs), which reduce inflammation in the gut and throughout the body.

The Med diet offers a long-term solution

One of the best things about the Med diet is that because it is tasty and varied, it is far easier to stick to than more restrictive diets.

- You don't eliminate lots of food groups.
- It's very adaptable and the principles can be applied to other cuisines.
- It's extremely filling, thanks to high-ish levels of fat, protein, and fiber in the diet.
- It is good for both your mental and your physical health.

Improving mental health is important, because many people give up trying to manage their weight when they become anxious or depressed.

In fact, a recent study of more than 33,000 people looked at the link between diet and depression and found that those who stuck closest to a traditional Mediterranean diet had a 33% lower risk of developing depression than those who didn't.[27]

Conversely, those who ate a typical "proinflammatory" diet, with lots of saturated fat, sugar, and processed food, had much higher rates of depression.

I certainly find that when I eat junk food it not only makes me miserable, but also makes me crave more.

More on this on page 140.

How does the Med diet compare with very low-carb diets, like keto and Atkins?

Studies like PREDIMED have shown that when it comes to your health, and your waist, the Med diet (which is moderately high in fat and low in carbs) is a much better option than going on a traditional low-fat diet. But how does it compare to really low-carb diets?

The keto diet, for example, is currently very fashionable. Like the Atkins diet, it is so low in carbs that your body is forced to "flip the metabolic switch," go into ketosis, and start burning fat for fuel. As I mentioned in Chapter 2, ketosis is also an important part of intermittent fasting. So, you may ask, why would one do the Med diet rather than one of these very low-carb diets?

Before trying to answer that I should explain what a keto diet is. There are variants, but a standard ketogenic diet is 75% fat, 20% protein, and just 5% carbs; which means you should aim to limit your carbs to less than 20g a day. To give you some context, a single banana has more than 20g of carbs.

Foods you can eat on a keto diet, or a very low-carb diet, like Atkins, include:

- Meat, bacon, sausages, fish, eggs, butter, cream, and cheese.
- Nuts, olive oil, coconut oil, and avocado oil.

- Fruits that are very low in carbs, such as berries.
- Leafy greens like spinach and broccoli.

You have to avoid:

- Anything with sugar in it, such as fruit juice, smoothies, or cake. This also includes many processed foods, takeout, and sauces.
- Bread, grains, rice, pasta, oats, and potatoes.
- Most fruits.
- Starchy vegetables such as sweet potatoes, carrots, and parsnips.
- Beans and legumes, such as lentils, chickpeas, kidney beans, and peas.
- Wine and beer. If you drink alcohol, it is best to stick to spirits.

A very low-carb diet like Atkins or keto can be a great way to lose weight, but it is also a diet which is hard to stick to, long term. The Med diet allows you to eat a much wider range of foods, including fruits, vegetables, and grains rich in the sort of fiber that will keep the "good" bacteria in your guts happy. It is hard to get the same variety of fiber and other essential nutrients if you are on an Atkins or keto diet. Not impossible, but hard.

So what would happen if you ran a scientific study comparing the Med diet with a low-carb diet like Atkins?

Well, a particularly impressive trial which did just that was carried out in Dimona, Israel, at a big research center with an on-site medical clinic. Unlike most diet studies, which tend to be short term, this one ran for more than six years.

The Dimona trial

For this study,[28] 322 middle-aged men and women were randomly assigned to a low-fat diet, a very low-carb diet (based on Atkins), or a lowish-carb Mediterranean diet. To take part you had to be 40–65 years old and have a BMI of at least 27 (i.e., overweight or obese).

Once they'd been recruited and allocated to a particular diet, the volunteers met up with a dietician who gave them advice on how to follow it. They had the usual tests before starting and at regular intervals throughout the trial.

For the first two years all the groups were good at sticking to their diets. They were also asked to keep diaries, which showed that:

- The Med-diet group ate the most fiber and the most olive oil.
- The low-carbers, not surprisingly, consumed the least carbs and the most fat and protein.
- The low-fat group cut their consumption of fat by an impressive 19%. They also cut their daily

calories by the greatest amount. But despite this they lost the least weight.

At the two-year mark, the results were an average weight loss of:

- 7.2 lb for the low-fat group
- 10 lb for the Med-diet group
- 11 lb for the low-carb group

So after two years it was the low-carbers, followed by the Med dieters, who were doing best in the weight-loss stakes, though it was the Med-diet group who saw the biggest improvements in their insulin levels.

But the study didn't stop there. They went on following the volunteers for another four years.

As you can imagine, I was agog to see these results because the key to any diet is whether you can keep it up long term. So what happened? Well, the low-fat and the low-carb dieters both put back on much of the weight they had lost. Those on the Med diet did not. Over the entire six-year period, the average weight loss was:

- 1.3 lb for the low-fat group
- 3.7 lb for the low-carb group
- 6.8 lb for the Med-diet group

In the long run, the clear winners were the Med dieters, who lost and kept off almost twice as much weight as the low-carbers. It is particularly impressive when you consider that over a six-year period a middle-aged person would normally expect to put on around 6.6 lb. In other words, at the end of six years, the group allocated to a Med-style diet actually weighed 13.2 lb less than you'd expect if they hadn't taken part in the trial.

As for health, when it came to cutting blood fats, "bad" cholesterol, insulin, and blood sugar levels, the undisputed winners were again the Med dieters. That's because they not only lost the most weight, they lost it in the right places.

In a related study,[29] involving lots of body scans, researchers found that it was Med dieters who lost the most fat around the waist, the heart, and inside the liver.

As Professor Iris Shai from Ben-Gurion University, who ran both studies, pointed out: "Even if you don't lose a lot of weight, going on a low-carb Mediterranean diet can have dramatic beneficial effects on fat deposits related to diabetes and cardiovascular diseases."

Q&A

What if I like eating other cuisines, like Indian or Thai?

The principles of the Med diet can be adapted to other cuisines, and you will see some examples in the recipe section. Olive oil, particularly extra-virgin, does seem to have an edge on other fats, but we also happily cook with coconut oil, and other nut oils like walnut. The main thing, if you are eating Indian, Chinese, or Thai, is to cut back on the rice and try to replace it with more vegetables. If you are a fan of Indian food, avoid the chapattis.

A variant on the Med diet is the Nordic diet, as eaten by Swedes, Danes, etc., in which olive oil is replaced with rapeseed oil. I'm not convinced that rapeseed oil is quite as good, but it's certainly better than the sort of junk food the rest of the world eats.

What if I'm a vegetarian or vegan?

The Med diet includes lots of vegetables and legumes, so it is well suited to a vegan or vegetarian lifestyle. Some of the recipes at the back of this book are vegetarian and some are vegan. And where possible we suggest tips and swaps for vegetarians.

To manage your substitutions it may be useful to download a calorie-counting app, such as My Fitness Pal. For example, coconut yogurt is higher in calories than dairy yogurt, so you will need to amend quantities. It is also important to consider that one of the valuable aspects of dairy yogurt is the variety of live cultures. If you are going to choose something to replace a yogurt recipe then it is really worth finding a substitute that has a good variety of live bacteria.

Isn't a Mediterranean diet expensive?

Fresh fish and extra-virgin olive oil are expensive, but so are all those sugary little treats and snacks that you will be cutting back on. A friend of mine who is an accountant, and who lost 66 lb on my diet, did a full spreadsheet and worked out that doing the diet actually saved him money.

A few money-saving tips:

- Extra-virgin olive oil for drizzling on salads can be expensive. But most supermarket brands are cheaper and virgin olive oil or light olive oil are good too.
- Fresh vegetables may be nicer, but there's not always much difference. Frozen or canned are just as nutritious.
- Try to eat berries such as strawberries and raspberries in season. Frozen berries are great for cooking.
- Apples and pears are normally quite cheap and long-lasting. We buy cooking apples when they are in season, and chop them and put them in the freezer. We never bother to peel them as that's where lots of the goodness lies.
- Canned or frozen fish is much cheaper than fresh fish, and lasts a lot longer.

- It is relatively easy to make your own live yogurt. All you need is milk and a dollop of fresh yogurt from a store-bought product. You can also use a yogurt-making machine.
- Fermented vegetables are very cheap to make and contain much higher levels of probiotics than the store-bought stuff. You can watch Clare making delicious sauerkraut at thefast800.com.
- Plain, unprocessed oatmeal is much cheaper than the instant stuff you buy in packets and much better for you.
- Making and taking your own lunch to work is going to be cheaper and healthier than dropping into the nearest sandwich bar.

5

GETTING ACTIVE

We all know how important it is to do exercise and remain active, but knowing something and doing it are very different things. I don't particularly like exercise, and I hate the gym, so I have found ways to make myself do what I need to do to keep myself healthy and happy, to sleep better, and keep my brain in decent shape.

Stand

The first and easiest thing you can do is stand every 30 minutes. Sitting continually is almost as bad as smoking. So get an app with an alarm that will remind you to move—every half an hour. If you watch a lot of TV, go for a stroll during the commercial breaks. Or keep the remote control beside the TV, so you have to get up to change channels.

Walk

Walking is a cheap and safe way to exercise and the best time to do it, if you can fit it into your life, is first thing in the morning, before breakfast. That way you not only manage to rev up your metabolism but you also get exposed to early morning light. Bright light in the morning helps reset your internal clock, which in turn will help you sleep better at night.

As for accessories, I would strongly recommend you take a friend or a loved one (I take the dog), but I wouldn't necessarily bother with an activity monitor.

In a myth-busting study,[30] researchers from the University of Pittsburgh recruited 470 overweight people aged 18 to 34 and asked them to lose weight on a low-calorie diet over a six-month period. Which they did. At the end of six months they were randomly allocated to either a standard behavioral program to help to keep the weight off or the same behavioral program plus an activity monitor. They were then followed for another 18 months.

At the end of this two-year trial there was a grand weigh-in. The group who were asked to wear the activity monitors were 7.7 lb lighter than at the start. Which was pretty good. Except that the group without the activity monitors had managed to keep off 13 lb, a lot more weight.

Why? The researchers didn't say, but I have a theory,

based on my behavior, which is that activity monitors not only encourage us to reward ourselves for hitting our targets by eating more, but they can also be depressing rather than motivating. You are forever trying to hit a target, such as the fabled "10,000 steps a day," which for many people is unachievable. So either you give up or you cheat.

To see if there is a better way to go, I got together with Professor Rob Copeland from Sheffield Hallam University. We collected a group of inactive volunteers and randomly allocated them to doing either 10,000 steps a day or going for what Professor Copeland called Active 10, three brisk 10-minute walks a day. Then we sent them on their way.

So what happened? Well, the group who were asked to do 10,000 steps a day really struggled to hit their target. They said they just couldn't fit it into their lives. The Active 10 group, on the other hand, got together in small walking groups, had more fun, and were much more likely to stick to their goals. Although the Active 10 walkers managed far fewer steps a day, when they were walking they were striding along much more intensely than those trying to hit 10,000 steps.

After analyzing their data, Professor Copeland pointed out to me that: "The Active 10 group spent 30% more time in the 'moderate to vigorous' physical activity zone, even though they were on the move for much less time. And that's important because it's when you are doing 'moderate to vigorous' activity that you get the greatest health benefits."

You can find a free app that will help guide you through Active 10 at www.nhs.uk/oneyou/active10/home.

HIIT

A few short, sharp bursts of brisk walking is a good way to start the day, but it isn't enough. If you like the idea of getting fitter but really don't feel you have the time, then you might want to try HIIT. With HIIT it really is possible to get most of the major benefits of exercise in very little time.

I first came across HIIT—high-intensity interval training—a few years ago while making a documentary called *The Truth about Exercise.*

Before starting, I was told that a few minutes a week of intense cycling would greatly improve my aerobic fitness and my blood sugar control. Which, to my great surprise, it did. The regimen I was asked to do consisted of three 20-second bursts of vigorous exercise on an exercise bike, three times a week. In just six weeks my insulin sensitivity improved by over 20%.

Since then Dr. Niels Vollaard, a lecturer in health and exercise science at the University of Stirling, has shown that you can get by on even less. It turns out that as little as 2 minutes of HIIT a week will give your body a significant boost.

In a recent experiment, which I helped Niels set up, we installed an exercise bike in the London office of Babylon, a health company, and asked some employees to try out five weeks of his HIIT regimen.

Before starting, Niels assessed their VO_2 max, a measure of aerobic fitness that shows how strong your heart and lungs are. He did these measurements in a lab, but you can get an estimate of yours by putting your resting heart rate into an online calculator, such as fast-exercises.com/fast-exercise-calculator.

This calculator will also tell you how you are doing for someone your age. For reasons we don't fully understand, VO_2 max is an incredibly powerful predictor of how well you are aging and your life expectancy. That's one of the main reasons why scientists such as Niels are so keen to find the most effective ways to improve it.

The attraction of HIIT is that it can produce the same sort of improvements in VO_2 max that you would get from much longer sessions of less vigorous activity. "To achieve the same results we get with HIIT," Niels told me, "you'd have to run at a decent pace for 45 minutes three times a week."

So what's going on? Niels says that when you do your first 20-second sprint your body breaks down glycogen, the form in which sugar is stored in your muscles. This sets off a cascade of other reactions, including the release of something he calls "signaling molecules."

When you do your next 20-second sprint, these signaling molecules are activated and help to stimulate the growth of other muscle, such as heart muscle. This, at least, is what has been shown to happen in the lab.

But would it also work in an office setting? Five weeks after the first set of tests, I returned with Niels to see how the office workers had gotten on. Most had managed to complete their ultrashort exercise regimen and most felt considerably fitter.

"We've analyzed the results," Niels told the volunteers, "and I am pleased to say that all of you improved. Our star performer, Charlie, improved his VO_2 max by 14%, while the group as a whole saw an improvement in fitness levels of 11%, which is excellent."

According to Niels, an 11% increase in aerobic fitness, if they kept it up, would mean a reduction in the risk of developing heart disease of about 20%.

HIIT isn't for everyone. If you're unfit then you should start slowly, doing just one 10-second sprint a session for the first week or so. If you are on medication, are injured, or have concerns about your heart, you should consult your doctor before starting any exercise regimen.

Dr. Vollaard's HIIT workout

To follow this regimen you will need an exercise bike on which you can easily vary the resistance. Do this three times a week.

1. Warm up with some gentle cycling.
2. After a minute or so begin pedaling fast, then swiftly crank up the resistance.
3. The level of resistance you select will depend on your strength and fitness. It should be high enough that, after 15 seconds of sprinting, your thighs begin to feel it and your muscles begin to fatigue.
4. If, after 15 seconds, you can keep going at the same pace, then the resistance you've chosen isn't high enough. It mustn't, however, be so high that you grind to a halt. It's a matter of experimenting. You'll find that as you get fitter the level of resistance you can cope with increases. Each 20-second workout should involve maximum effort.
5. After your first burst of fast sprinting, drop the resistance and do 3 minutes of gentle pedaling.
6. Then do the 20-second sprint again.
7. Finish with a couple of minutes of gentle cycling to allow your heart rate and blood pressure to return to normal before stepping off the bike.

If you are a total beginner to HIIT I would start by doing just one 20-second burst and see how you feel. You can gradually build it up from there.

I still do my 3 × 20-seconds regimen, three times a week. In a recent American study,[31] they got 27 sedentary overweight men to do 3 × 20-second sessions of HIIT three times a week for 12 weeks and found that this not only improved their VO_2 max by 19%, but also increased their insulin sensitivity. HIIT produced similar results to cycling briskly for 45 minutes, three times a week, but took a fraction of the time.

Without a bike it is harder to do a HIIT session, although you can swap cycling for running up stairs for 20 seconds or putting in short, flat-out sprints when jogging. You can also do it while swimming. Again, it is just a 20-second burst.

Strength training

As well as looking after your heart and lungs, you also need to look after your muscles. Muscles look good on the beach, but more important, they burn calories even when you are sleeping. Improving your muscles will also improve your insulin sensitivity.

I have a simple regimen, which I do most mornings. I get out of bed, put the radio on, and do a series of push-ups, squats, abdominal crunches, the bicep curl and the plank—in roughly this order. There are lots of other variants you can try, but these are the basics. Again, if you want to see how they should be done, visit thefast800.com.

I suggest you start by doing one set of 10 repeats

of each of these in Week 1 of the diet (with 20-second holds on the planks). In other words: 10 push-ups, 10 crunches, 10 squats. Do this three times in the first week. Aim for two sets of 10 repeats by Week 2, and three sets by Week 4.

12 ways to introduce more activity into your life

1. Buy a bike and cycle when you can. It saves lots of time and money.
2. If your destination is less than a mile away, then why not walk? It will take you less time than waiting for a bus or finding somewhere to park.
3. Stand while talking on the phone. You'll burn calories and sound more assertive.
4. Use a basket at the shops rather than a shopping cart. That way you do a bit of resistance training while shopping.
5. Drink lots of water. This not only keeps you hydrated but also increases the need for bathroom breaks, which means in turn more short, brisk walks.
6. Try, where possible, to take the stairs. I always run up escalators.
7. If you normally take a bus or train to work, get off at an earlier stop than usual and walk the rest of the way.

8. If you drive to work or the supermarket, park at the far end of the car park.

9. Keep resistance bands—stretchy cords or tubes that offer resistance when you pull on them— or small hand weights near your desk. Do arm curls between meetings or tasks.

10. Organize a lunchtime walking group. You might be surrounded by people who are just dying to lace up their sneakers. Enjoy the camaraderie, and offer encouragement to one another when you feel like giving up.

11. If I am on vacation in a foreign city, I normally join a two-hour guided walking tour. They are cheap and a great introduction to a city's history. The one I went on in Berlin was particularly good.

12. Go to dancing classes. It is sociable and if you haven't ever learned how to do classic steps, like Latin or ballroom, it will be mentally challenging. Taking up a new challenge in middle age is a proven way to cut your risk of dementia.

6

WAYS TO BEAT STRESS

Many of us feel bad about putting on weight because we think it is entirely our own fault. After all, we have been told time and time again that the only reason anyone packs on those extra pounds is that they are eating too much and not doing enough exercise. In other words, if we get fat it must be because we are greedy and idle.

As we've already seen, weight gain is nothing like as simple as that. The foods we eat (processed and heavily promoted by the food industry) can hijack our brains and our hormones, while the world we live in has been built to discourage activity. Shopping centers are increasingly out of town and only accessible by car. Roads are dangerous to cycle on and, though elevators are easy to find, stairs are not.

We are surrounded by constant temptation, which is hard to resist. What the "calories in, calories out" crowd also ignore is the overwhelming importance of stress. Research has shown that chronic stress leads to

114

increased hunger, comfort eating, self-loathing, and disrupted sleep. This, in turn, leads to even higher levels of stress, and more hunger, eating, self-loathing, etc.

What is stress?

You need some level of stress in your life. It is essential for survival. If you are crossing the road and realize you are in the path of a car, your body will release huge amounts of stress hormones, such as cortisol and adrenaline, to ready you for physical action. This is the "fight-or-flight" response, and it evolved because in the distant past it would have helped us avoid being eaten by predators. This is a good thing. The problem is long-term stress, when levels of these stress hormones go up and stay up.

How stress and insomnia fuel your hunger

There are lots of things that life throws at us that we can't control: losing a job, getting divorced, losing a loved one, having an accident. All of these are serious setbacks which can cause deep stress and, in turn, trigger comfort eating. The techniques I'm about to describe won't reduce the immediate pain, but they may help reduce the impact of these life events.

That said, there is one major stress inducer which

you can and should look at in your life—lack of sleep. Insomnia is common and often self-induced; "self-induced" in the sense that we stay up late on social media and don't prioritize sleep.

And yet skimping on sleep is one of the worst things you can do if you are trying to lose weight or keep it off. Even a couple of nights when you cut back on sleep can play havoc with your blood sugars and your hunger hormones.

To test this out, I joined Dr. Eleanor Scott, of Leeds University, in a short, sharp sleep-deprivation experiment. For this experiment, Dr. Scott recruited a group of healthy volunteers and fitted them with glucose monitors, so that she could see what was happening to their blood sugar levels. She asked the volunteers to go to bed two hours later than normal for two nights, then to sleep as long as they liked for two nights.

Naturally enough, being an avid self-experimenter, I joined in. The two nights when we went to bed two hours late were pretty grim. I was also unpleasantly surprised by just how much my blood sugar levels rose on the days when I was sleep-deprived, and how hungry I was.

The same was true for all my fellow volunteers—everyone complained about having had the munchies when they had less sleep. As one of them told me: "I wanted lots of cookies and I didn't just have one—I had 10 custard creams."

"Is that unusual?" I asked him.

"Well, it is certainly unusual for breakfast!" he replied.

All of us, whether we had feasted on cookies or managed to stick to our normal diet, saw big increases in our blood sugar levels, to the point where previously healthy individuals had levels you would see in type 2 diabetics. Fortunately, these problems were resolved after a couple of nights of good sleep.

So it is not surprising that being sleep-deprived leads to overeating. A study by researchers at King's College, London,[32] found that if you deprive people of sleep, they consume, on average, an extra 385 calories per day, which is the equivalent of a large muffin.

Ways to beat stress and anxiety

- Losing weight will mean that you sleep better, which means you will be less likely to feel those sleep-deprived bingeing urges.
- Intermittent fasting, like the 5:2, has been shown to improve mood, probably by boosting levels of the hormone BDNF (see page 56).
- Among the many benefits of eating a Mediterranean-style diet are the effects on your brain. Studies by the Food and Mood Centre in Australia[33] have shown that going on a Med diet can have a big impact on anxiety and depression.

In one study they found that 12 weeks on a Mediterranean diet was enough to significantly improve the mood of people suffering from severe anxiety or depression.

- No one knows exactly why this is, but some of the components (such as the fish and the olive oil) have a well-established anti-inflammatory effect, and there is mounting evidence that many cases of depression may be linked to inflammation caused by the body's immune system reacting to infection or stress.

- Exercise is also a great stress-buster. It pumps up the production of your brain's feel-good neuro-transmitters, including BDNF and endorphins. It gets you out of yourself—and can also improve your sleep, which as we've just seen has a direct impact on mood.

Mindfulness

As well as all of the above, I would recommend you take up mindfulness. There are lots of different approaches, including taking a course, but the one I do is a guided meditation via an app. I do it for 5–10 minutes most mornings. Try doing the following brief routine, just to get a flavor: sit in a comfortable chair, rest your hands on your thighs, close your eyes, then for the next few minutes try to focus on your breath.

1. Breathe in to a count of four through your nose and then, without pausing or holding your breath, let the air flow out gently, counting from one to four.
2. Keep doing this for 3–5 minutes.

Try to pay attention to the sensation of your breath going through your nostrils, filling your chest, expanding and contracting your diaphragm. Try to stay focused on the task, and when you notice that your thoughts have drifted, which they will, gently bring them back to your breath. It is surprisingly hard to do, but like any form of exercise it gets easier.

It is also a good way of drifting off to sleep if you feel like your thoughts are keeping you awake.

You might also want to try a few of the following exercises. These are courtesy of a friend of mine, Tim Stead, who teaches at the Oxford Mindfulness Centre and has written a terrific book called *See, Love, Be*.

The raisin practice

This is a classic. It doesn't have to be done with a raisin, but it seems to work particularly well with raisins.

1. Take a raisin and place it on the palm of your hand.
2. Now just inspect the raisin. Study the texture, the colors, the way that light plays on its surface.

Then pick it up and roll it around between your fingers. Squish it a bit. Smell it. Admire it.

3. Put the raisin on your tongue and taste it. Notice the way that your mouth fills with saliva in anticipation of the treat to come.

4. When you are ready, bite into it and notice how the flavors are released. Where in the mouth can you really taste that raisin? How would you describe it?

5. Finally, swallow the raisin.

You can do the same sort of thing with a cup of coffee, a bite of apple . . . any food or drink. It is all about taking a few moments to really savor the experience.

The kindness practice

To do this, find somewhere quiet and comfortable to sit, and then say this phrase in your head several times: "May I be kept safe and may I know kindness."

It can feel awkward to begin with, but it is a way of cultivating an attitude of kindness toward yourself. We spend so much time listening to that little voice in our heads that is endlessly critical. This is one way to strike back.

The prodigal son practice

First thing in the morning, set your cell phone alarm for some random time in the day. When it goes off stop what you are doing and look around.

Notice where you are, who else is around, what thoughts were going through your mind when the alarm went. Ask yourself what your mood is like. How are you feeling?

Check in with your body. How's the knee? Think about what you would like to do next—not what you always do, perhaps something different. The point of this exercise is to shake up your normal routine and make you realize you have choices.

Mindfulness in nature

Gardening is a great way to get some exercise and reduce stress, but you don't need a garden to do this particular mental exercise. Just go outside or to a nearby park. Find some flowers and look at them. Really look at them. You don't need to know their name; you are just choosing a moment to admire their colors, their patterns, the way they grow.

As you do this your mind will wander. You will start thinking about what you need to do next or what you are going to have for your next meal. Try to keep coming back to the flowers. Just for a few minutes.

Mindfulness is not a panacea and it certainly doesn't work for everyone. Vulnerable people, such as those with post-traumatic stress disorder, should be particularly careful before undertaking mindfulness. That said, most people who stick with it do benefit.

7

THE FAST800 IN PRACTICE

The Fast800 has three stages: Rapid Weight Loss, the New 5:2, and Maintenance. I am not going to be prescriptive about how long you stay in the first two stages because that depends entirely on how much weight you want to lose and whether you are finding that particular stage easy to stick to.

Although I recommend you start with Rapid Weight Loss, it won't suit everyone. You can use it to kick-start things, and after a few weeks move on to 5:2. Or you may find you are getting such great results you want to go on for a while.

On the next pages I offer a brief outline of the three stages and how they work. I then go into more detail about what to expect and how to fit the diet into your life.

Stage 1: The Very Fast800—rapid weight loss

For the Rapid Weight Loss stage of the diet, you eat 800 calories a day. I suggest you stay on this stage for a minimum of two weeks, but you can stay on it for anything up to 12 weeks, depending on your circumstances and how much weight you have to lose.

To make up your 800 calories, you can either rely on the menus in this book, or use meal replacement shakes if you find them easier. I know that 800 calories doesn't sound like a lot, but the menus are designed to be filling as well as nutrient-rich.

Because it is a low-carb as well as low-calorie diet, it should induce mild ketosis (which you can use urine sticks to check). This will take a few days to kick in.

As your body switches from burning sugar to burning fat, it will produce ketones, which will help suppress your appetite. But because you are not used to this you may get headaches or become light-headed. These symptoms may be due to dehydration and should pass. More on side effects and how to counter them later.

As well as cutting down to 800 calories a day, I recommend adding in a Time Restricted Eating (TRE) program. This means, from the start, aiming for a 12-hour overnight fast. More on how to do this on page 139.

Stage 2: The New 5:2—intermittent fasting

At some point, it may be at the end of the first two weeks or it may be later (depending on how you get on), you are going to want to switch from the Rapid Weight Loss phase to something which is more gradual. This means switching from 800 calories every day to intermittent fasting, where you will be on 800 calories for a few days a week.

On the days when you are not fasting, you don't have to count calories, though you will need to be careful about portion control and maintain a superhealthy Mediterranean-style diet (see the recipes at the back of this book).

At this stage I'd suggest you try extending your overnight fast by reducing your TRE window from 12 hours to 10 hours. In other words, making your overnight fast last 14 hours. The reason for doing this is that it will help maintain and enhance the benefits of intermittent fasting, in particular autophagy and ketosis.

Stage 3. Maintenance—a way of life

Once you've achieved your goals it will be time to go on to the Maintenance Phase. This will be another hugely important moment, a time when you consolidate all the things you have learned, but also a time where you might be tempted to go back to your previous habits. The good news is that the longer you stick to the maintenance program, the easier and more natural it becomes.

The Fast800 at a glance:

	How to fast	What to eat	When to eat
Stage 1. **Rapid Weight** **Loss**	800 calories a day for up to 12 weeks	Real food (see recipes) or meal replacement shakes	TRE 12:12
Stage 2. **The New 5:2**	800 calories, 2 days a week	On 800 days: real food (see recipes) or shakes. On nonfast days: Med-style diet with portion control	TRE 10:14 or 16:8
Stage 3. **Maintenance**	No calorie counting, though you might do a weekly fast day—6:1	Healthy Med-style diet	TRE 12:12 or 10:14

BEFORE YOU START

I've tried to make this diet as simple and doable as possible. It is based on solid science. But before you get going I want you to be sure that this is the right approach for you. Going on the Fast800 will have a powerful and beneficial impact on your weight and metabolism, but it won't suit everyone. So do go back and look at who should and shouldn't do the rapid weight-loss stage (see page 85).

Tests and targets

Getting to know your body before you start the diet is important, not just to ensure that it is suitable and safe for you, but because it will help to keep you motivated and focused on what you are hoping to achieve.

If you are significantly overweight, or have other medical conditions, you may need to enlist your health professional's support in monitoring and motivating you along the way.

Basic measurements that you can do at home:

WWR: Weight, Waist, and Resting Heart Rate

- Step on the scale and weigh yourself, ideally first thing in the morning before eating or drinking.

- Measure your waist around your belly button.
- Measure your resting heart rate first thing, before doing exercise.
- Keep a record of your results.

More sophisticated home measurements

A **blood sugar monitor** will show if you have prediabetes or diabetes. It involves pricking your finger and measuring blood sugar levels. Over 30% of the adult population have prediabetes (raised blood sugars which are not yet in the diabetic range) and unless you have been tested it is extremely unlikely that you will know. One in four people with type 2 diabetes are also unaware that they have it.

You can buy a blood sugar monitor from a pharmacy or online. It is a useful device even if you don't have raised blood sugar levels because it will show you how your body responds to different foods. When we tested ourselves, Clare and I both discovered that bread and white rice send our blood sugars soaring.

Another thing you might want to try are **ketone test strips,** which you can also buy online. The ones that rely on blood prick tests are more accurate, but the urine sticks are cheaper and simpler.

Nutritional ketosis is a natural and desirable side effect of fasting. Note that it is very different from Diabetic Keto Acidosis (DKA), a serious complication seen in diabetics with dangerously high levels of ketones.

There are also various medical tests that you might find useful, but these are not essential. For information on these, please see page 269.

Be clear about your GOALS:

Once you've done the measurements and tests you will have a better idea of what it is you want to achieve. You may discover, for example, that you are prediabetic and want to get your blood sugars back to normal. Maybe you are fairly healthy but with a bit too much visceral fat. Or perhaps you simply want to fit into some favorite old clothes.

Get: What do you want to get out of this diet? Weight loss? Better blood sugars? A smaller waist? To come off medication?

Opportunities: What resources and opportunities are available to help you succeed? Friends and family? Professionals? Diet buddy? An online forum like the one at www.thefast800.com?

Approach: How do you intend to approach this diet? What steps do you need to take to help you succeed? What has worked in the past? What will help keep you on track? Which combination of 800-calorie days could work for you?

Look for successes: Take one day at a time—look for small changes in your measurements, how you feel, your energy levels, your activity levels. Notice and celebrate small positive changes.

Use a notebook to record your goals. It helps to make a list of what you want to achieve and how you plan to achieve it—laminate it and stick it on the fridge, or the bathroom mirror or door. Remembering why you are doing the diet will really help in those moments of weakness, when motivation is faltering.

Clear out the cupboards!

Willpower is hugely overrated and relying on it is one of the main reasons why so many diets fail. Old habits are hard to break. The way to succeed is to create an environment in which it is easier to succeed than to fail.

So before you start, rid your house of junk food. This is like "autophagy," clearing out the junky old cells to make space for new ones. There is a lot of truth behind the saying "out of sight, out of mind." It's just too hard to resist "treat" food if it's right in front of you.

Foods to give away, hide, or throw out include:

1. Most breakfast cereals, as they are processed and sugary (apart from plain oats).
2. Sugary cakes, cookies, and sweets.
3. Chocolate (apart from dark chocolate with over 70% cocoa content).
4. Snacks, including breakfast/snack bars, chips, and dried fruit.

5. Ready-made meals and canned soups (often high in added sugar).
6. Breads, flatbreads, and crackers.
7. Sweet tropical fruit.
8. Juices, cordials, smoothies, and sugary soft drinks.
9. Alcohol.

Getting rid of this food is easier if everyone in the house is happy to have it gone. If you have young kids or a partner who isn't doing the diet, I recommend that you get them and any other household members to hide all "treat" foods from you.

You could even ask them to keep the treats in a locked or hidden cupboard and make sure you have no access to the key. Crazy, but when you are desperate you will go looking. Believe me, I've been there. You have to think of junk food as being like crack cocaine. You wouldn't keep it in the house.

Ten healthy foods to stock your fridge and cupboards with:

Once you've gotten rid of the junk it's time to restock. Having no food in the house is almost as bad as having lots of junk food. You will end up eating takeout or dropping into the gas station to buy snacks. Here are

10 essentials, many of which will be useful for making the recipes at the back of the book.

1. **A large bottle of olive oil.** Be generous with it. Use olive oil or unprocessed/virgin rapeseed oil when cooking. And get a bottle of extra-virgin olive oil to use in salads.

2. **Vegetables**—lots of them, particularly spinach, broccoli, kale, carrots, bell peppers, eggplant, tomatoes, cucumbers, and zucchini. Precut some carrots, celery, or cucumber to snack on if you feel you really need something. Put them at the top of the fridge where you will see them when you open the fridge door.

3. **Fruit.** Fruit is a great alternative to cakes and cookies if you feel like something sweet, but limit it to two pieces a day and eat it after a meal rather than as a snack as it stops ketosis—i.e., fat burning. Stick to lower-sugar fruits such as berries, apples, and pears.

4. **Full-fat dairy products**—such as full-fat live Greek yogurt, cheese, and butter. Healthy natural fats will keep you full for longer. When I need a snack it is a small chunk of cheese with some slices of pear.

5. **Unsalted and unsweetened nuts and seeds**. Aim for a variety, such as almonds, cashews, Brazil nuts, walnuts, sunflower seeds, pine nuts, chia and sesame seeds. Roast them, to enhance the flavor, and store them in a jar. Nuts are rich in fiber to feed your microbiome and an excellent source of healthy natural fat. But eat no more than a small handful.

6. **Whole grains**—such as brown and wild rice, quinoa, or pearl barley. Small amounts of these can be added to your meals instead of white rice and pasta. Try to cut out bread completely. It is hard, but "going brown" is unlikely to reduce the sugar hit. Have the occasional slice of seeded whole grain bread or dark rye bread if you must.

7. **Eggs**. We always have eggs on standby and have them for breakfast most days of the week. They are a great source of protein and will keep you feeling fuller for longer. My kids eat them raw! (I'm told it is a body-building thing.)

8. **Oily fish**. Smoked salmon goes well with eggs for breakfast and canned tuna can be a great snack or lunchtime alternative. Smoked mackerel is super easy to prepare and full of flavor. Aim to eat oily fish 2–3 times a week.

9. **Beans and lentils.** Dried, canned, or precooked in packets, legumes are rich in vegetable protein and nutrients. They usually taste best when sprinkled with olive oil. Sneak a handful into stews, salads, and bakes. They are an excellent source of fiber, essential for a healthy microbiome.

10. **Fizzy water and herbal teas.** Soda water can help to ease hunger pangs without adding calories. Include a piece of lemon, lime, or cucumber for flavor. Herbal teas are another useful alternative to sugary drinks. You'll find a wide range of flavors in most supermarkets. Keep cold herbal tea in the fridge.

Broadcast the news

Don't keep it a secret. Tell your friends and family you are going on this diet and that you need them to be supportive. Ultimately, *you* have control over what you eat, but it helps if a friend isn't encouraging you to have a piece of cake with your coffee. If people know you are on this diet, they will be considerate about what they eat around you and won't offer you "treat" foods or put temptation your way.

It is vital that the people close to you understand

why you are doing this diet and what you want to achieve. Encourage them to try out the recipes with you—they don't have to stick to 800 calories per day (many of the recipes have tips for how to adapt them for nonfast days), but the more you can do together, the better. Talking about nutrition with others will really cement your understanding of how different foods can affect your health.

Q & A

Should I start by doing 800 calories every day?

The first decision you need to make is whether you want to start with the Very Fast800 or the New 5:2. This depends on your motivation and how much weight you want to lose. The advantage of the Very Fast800 is, of course, that the weight loss will be dramatic and that can be very motivating, but you need to be sure you are comfortable about trying. I suggest that you commit to this stage for two weeks, then reassess (see below).

Should I start off with real food or with meal replacement diet shakes?

Some people think that using meal replacement diet shakes is "cheating," others find it really helps, particularly at the start, because then you don't have to think about what to buy and cook for every meal. It also means you don't have to worry about counting calories or getting in all your essential nutrients for those meals. Plus they can be a quick and easy solution when dashing out first thing in the morning or to take to work for lunch.

I'm very pragmatic about this. If you would prefer to try to do the Very Fast800 with real food, that's what the menus in this book are for. If, instead, you would like to replace some of your meals with shakes then do visit our website, thefast800.com, where I suggest a number of different brands which are more suited to a low-carb Mediterranean style of eating.

Unfortunately, a lot of meal replacement shakes contain added sugar, taste artificial, and are surprisingly high in carbs. If you want to go the shake route, you should aim for something low in carbs, and containing plenty of protein, enough fat, and decent amounts of fiber.

Should I take a vitamin supplement?

The menus in this book are designed to ensure that you get all the necessary minerals and vitamins. Nonetheless, you may, as a precaution, want to try a reputable brand, particularly on fast days, and perhaps also fish oil supplements.

STAGE 1—WHAT TO EXPECT

Just to remind you, if you have decided to kick off with the Very Fast800, you are going to be sticking to 800 calories a day, every day, for at least the next two weeks. This will lead to some impressive changes, which many people find extremely motivating. And remember, as I've mentioned before, the amount of weight you lose early on is a great predictor of how much you will lose overall.

Managing the first two weeks

The first week or two are likely to be the toughest, as your body adapts to fewer calories and to "flipping the metabolic switch." Your body will be burning more fat and less sugar, which is good, but this can produce side effects. During this time you are also getting used to eating and preparing food differently. So it is likely to feel like quite a challenge on all fronts.

That said, most people find sticking to 800 calories a day eminently manageable and are astonished that the hunger soon passes.

A friend of mine, Dick, who went on this diet to reverse his type 2 diabetes, lost 15.4 lb in the first two weeks and 30.8 lb in just eight weeks. Three years later, he's not only kept the weight off but his blood sugars remain completely normal, without medication (much to his doctor's surprise).

What's his secret? "I eat the things that I really love, like pasta, but in small portions. I keep a close track of my weight and I don't allow it to creep up. The most weight I ever put on is 2 or 3 lb over Christmas and I make sure I get rid of it straight afterward."

Side effects

When you do the Fast800 you will, like Dick, begin to lose a lot of weight, fast. Some of it will be fat, but initially you will also be passing a lot of urine. Unless you keep topping yourself up with fluid this may leave you feeling light-headed, tired, headachy.

This is why I encourage people to drink lots of fluid. Try adding a little salt to food, especially if you don't normally use salt. Taking a supplement that contains magnesium, potassium, and B vitamins can also help.

What you drink is up to you, as long as it doesn't contain calories. Tap water is fine. I prefer it cooled from the fridge. I also love fizzy water with a little lemon. Fruit tea is good, too, and you can have the occasional coffee (but only a splash of milk, if any). Some people like plain hot water, and oddly enough there is evidence that heat alone can soothe hunger. Zero-calorie fizzy drinks if you must. But no fruit juice or smoothies.

How to introduce TRE (Time Restricted Eating)

Do give TRE a go. I would start by trying to fit your 800 calories into a 12-hour window, which probably means having a slightly later breakfast and an earlier evening meal in order to extend your normal night-time fast. I found that when I did this (see page 66) it actually made the whole diet easier.

The main problem with having a later breakfast is that you may struggle to find suitable low-calorie eating options near your place of work. In that case you might want to take your breakfast (or a meal replacement shake) with you to eat at work. Remember, you can drink as much water, black tea, herbal tea, and black coffee as you want when you wake. It is only food or drink which contains calories that you need to avoid.

Spend a couple of weeks getting used to eating within a 12-hour period before trying to reduce your eating window further.

Doing exercise

If you already have a regular exercise program, just keep going. If you don't do regular exercise, this is a good time to begin. Start by doing a few brisk walks (ideally in the morning light, before breakfast) and some light resistance exercises, such as push-ups and squats. These should increase in frequency and intensity as the weeks go by. Doing exercise will improve your sleep and will help push you into ketosis faster, which in turn means you will be increasing the effectiveness of the diet. You shouldn't use exercise as an excuse to eat more and you shouldn't use the fact you are on a diet as an excuse to stop exercising. Be sensible. If you are planning on running the marathon some time in the next few weeks, don't start fasting just beforehand.

How to deal with cravings

The first two weeks are when you will feel the strongest cravings. After this they will diminish—truly! Here's a quick checklist to help boost your resolve.

1. Remove temptation—again. Have you definitely done this? Removing tempting treats from the house will make resisting cravings so much easier (see page 130).

2. Remember why you are doing this. This is why it is so important that you have clear goals (see page 129). One of the great things about the Fast800 is that people see and feel big changes really quickly. If you feel tempted to have that cake or that bit of toast then pause, breathe in and out a few times, and think of those clothes you will be able to wear or the relief of hearing that your blood sugars have returned to normal—and generally how you are going to feel at the end of the program.

3. Try to understand why you are craving something. Are you bored? Are you actually thirsty rather than hungry? Perhaps you are feeling tired and just need to put your feet up briefly? I find that when I'm tired or stressed my first instinct is to reach for a snack to reduce the discomfort. Instead, distract yourself.

4. Say to yourself "it will pass!" Going for a brisk walk or reading a magazine will often help shift your mind onto something else. Sip an herbal tea. Sing. It will pass.

5. Use meal replacement shakes. If you are finding the whole process of following recipes and calorie counting just too tough at first, replace some of your meals with shakes while you get in the groove.

6. Make the most of your backup support. At some point you are bound to hear that sneaky inner voice that tries to justify a break in your diet. "It's just this once." This is when we are at our most vulnerable. And when it is most important to rely on your support systems to help you avoid temptation and steer clear of "saboteurs."

On the other hand, if you do give in, don't use that as an excuse to give up altogether. Just get back on the horse and keep riding.

After the first two weeks—questions to ask yourself

After two weeks is a good time to assess how things are going. Is the diet doing what you hoped it would do? How are you feeling, and are you coping?

If you are feeling fine, then do keep going. In the DIRECT study and the DROPLET trial, most people stuck to 800 calories a day for 8–12 weeks, but this very much depends on how you feel.

1. *Are you losing weight?* By the end of Week 2 the rate at which you are losing weight may have slowed but it should still be rapid. Based on clinical trials, average weight loss at the end of Week 2 should be around 8.8 lb if you are doing the Very Fast800, 3.3 lb if you are doing 5:2.

    If you are not losing much weight, check that you are actually sticking to the 800 calories and that you're not slipping in the occasional snack! The recipes at the back of this book will show you what 800 calories looks like.

    By now you should be in nutritional ketosis. It is worth checking that you are producing

142

ketones (using ketone test strips). If not, you may need to reduce your carbs more to achieve it. How low you need to go varies from one person to another.

2. *Is your appetite under better control?* Most people report feeling less hungry by the end of Week 2 and that their cravings are weaker. If you are still feeling hungry much of the time, check you are eating at least 50–60g of protein a day. Lack of protein is one of the major drivers of hunger.

3. *Are you feeling light-headed or feeble?* This can happen as people adapt to burning ketones. It is sometimes called "keto flu." Symptoms include mood swings, irritability, and dizziness. Like the flu, it will pass.

   If you are not already taking a supplement, I would recommend one containing decent amounts of magnesium, potassium, and vitamins B and D. Low levels of any of these are linked to fatigue.

   You may simply be dehydrated. You should be drinking enough water to pass at least 5–6 good volumes of urine a day.

   It goes without saying that if you are experiencing more severe symptoms, such as fever, vomiting, or frequent and/or prolonged diarrhea, you should stop the diet immediately and contact your doctor.

4. *Are you getting constipated?* If so I would recommend not only drinking extra fluids, but also adding more fiber-rich food, such as non-starchy vegetables—leafy greens, spinach, kale, broccoli, cauliflower—as well as blackberries, chia seeds, or flaxseeds. You may consider getting something from the pharmacy such as a natural soluble fiber or an osmotic laxative, which draws more fluid into the gut, softening the stool.

5. *Are you sleeping?* If not, you may wish to eat your main meal a bit later, increase your activity levels, get outside in the daylight every day, twice if possible. This resets your internal clock and improves your mood.

6. *Are you getting bad breath?* Some people start producing the sweet fruity smell of ketones on their breath. It's a bit like nail polish remover. This is normal and shows the diet is working. Brush your teeth regularly and press on!

7. *How is your mood? Are you coping?* You may sometimes feel irritable and "hangry" but I would be concerned about a prolonged drop in

mood. If this is the case, do talk to someone or seek professional advice.

If you are finding the diet too tough . . .

If, for example, you are having frequent lapses, you may want to consider slowing things down a bit:

- Some people find it easier to do 2:5. You fast during the week and eat healthily at the weekend without worrying too much about the calories (but sticking to the principles of the Med diet).
- You might want to switch to the New 5:2 approach, fasting two days a week and eating healthily on the other days (see page 125).
- Or you might want to have a total break from dieting. Counterintuitive though it sounds, having a regular break from dieting, "intermittent dieting," can be more effective than just plowing on, as the Matador study showed.

Intermittent dieting: the Matador study

For this study,[34] 51 obese men were randomly allocated to either a constant low-calorie diet for 16 weeks, or the same diet done in stages.

Those who were allocated to what was called

"intermittent dieting" were asked to diet for two weeks, then return to balanced eating for two weeks, then diet for another two weeks, etc. They did this for 30 weeks, so that in total they did 16 weeks of actual dieting, the same number as the constant dieters.

Both groups were measured at the beginning and end of the experiment, then six months later.

So what happened? Well, at the end of the first stage of the experiment the regular dieters had lost an average of 19.8 lb, while the intermittent dieters had lost an average of 30.8 lb.

When they were tested again, six months later, the steady dieters had put back on most of the weight, while the intermittent dieters had not.

The final figures were an average weight loss of 6.6 lb for the constant dieters versus 24.2 lb for the intermittent dieters. In other words, doing intermittent dieting made an impressive 17.6 lb difference.

Why? It's possible that doing a diet in stages helps beat dieting fatigue. The researchers also found that those who followed a "two weeks on, two weeks off" dieting pattern not only lost more weight, but lost more fat and preserved more muscle too. Which led to a smaller drop in their metabolic rate.

By the end of the diet the men who had been asked to do intermittent dieting were burning an average of 92 more calories a day than those who had lost equal amounts of weight through constant dieting. One of the lead researchers, Professor Amanda Sainsbury-Salis, from the University of Sydney, told me that intermittent dieting was the way she herself had lost weight. "I would restrict for as long as I could handle it, which was usually for around two weeks, sometimes 10 days, then take a break of a few weeks before dieting again."

This was a relatively small trial, designed to test out this novel approach, and it was only conducted with men. A team from the University of Tasmania is currently doing a bigger study with women, with results expected sometime in 2019.

STAGE 2: SWITCHING TO THE NEW 5:2.

Once you have kick-started your weight loss with the Very Fast800 you are on a roll. It is entirely up to you when you move on to Stage 2, the New 5:2—some of you will find a couple of weeks' rapid weight loss enough; others will want to stay on Stage 1 for longer, depending on your goals. But either way your hunger levels and your cravings should be much reduced. You should also find you are feeling more energetic, lighter, and brighter. People will have begun to comment on how well you are looking.

Switching over is straightforward and can be done at any point that suits you. For the 800-calorie fast days, you continue to use the low-calorie recipes in this book (or, if you prefer, a mix of meal replacement shakes and real food). On the other days, you can eat normally, but healthily, i.e., sticking to a Med-style diet, low in carbs and refined sugars, without counting calories.

How to choose your 800-calorie days

I am often asked whether it is better, when doing the 5:2, to do your 800-calorie days back-to-back or split. In theory you might be better off doing them back-to-back because that way you will get into ketosis on the first day, then stay in ketosis for the whole of the second day. Some people also find it more convenient to get their fasting over and done with in one go. Others, however, prefer to do split days. In the end you have to find what works for you. The main thing is that when you have chosen your days, you should try to stick with them. Changing your fast days means you are less likely to do them.

When to eat your calories on an 800-calorie day

We are all different. When I'm doing the 5:2, I prefer eating my calories in just two meals, while putting aside some calories for a small snack. I have a late breakfast, skip lunch, and aim to eat early in the evening. As you can see from our menus, we offer you choices. You can have three smallish meals—breakfast, lunch, and dinner—or spread your calories over two larger meals. Try the different approaches till you the find one that works for you.

What to eat on nonfast days

We have included "nonfast day" options at the end of many of our recipes to make it easier for you to follow a healthy diet even on the "normal" days. There are suggestions for how to include extras such as added protein (see page 243) or to add in whole grains (such as brown rice or quinoa), lentils, and beans. You can sometimes include a slice of brown seeded or sourdough bread, and even the occasional dessert after a meal, or a portion of fruit. For some recipes you can simply double the portions. There are also suggestions as to how to make the recipe a bit more substantial, perhaps by adding extra nonstarchy vegetables or a dressed salad.

How to combine the New 5:2 with TRE

If you have been following a Time Restricted Eating plan you can either stick to your current regimen (which will either be 12:12 or 14:10) or you can move on to something a little bit tougher, which is 16:8. Just to remind you, this means not eating or drinking anything which contains calories for 16 hours, overnight.

As we saw in Chapter 3, fasting for longer will deliver more powerful benefits, but it can be harder to stick to.

One of the most common ways that people do the 16:8 is by skipping breakfast and not eating until at least 12 p.m. Before that time you can have black tea, black coffee, plenty of water, but no actual calories. If you are serious about doing TRE then do try to eat your last calories at least three hours before going to bed.

Again, in the evenings, when you have stopped eating, you can have as many calorie-free drinks as you want—water, herbal teas, and so on—but, obviously, no alcohol!

In fact, my advice is that you try to lower or even cut out alcohol altogether while trying to lose weight. Alcohol is bad for dieters for a range of reasons:

- It weakens your willpower—I find that once I've had a drink, my willpower, always weak to begin with, almost entirely disappears.
- Alcohol gives you the munchies. When I am drinking I cannot resist crisps.
- Alcohol is extremely caloric. Here are a few figures to bear in mind: a large glass of wine (8.4 oz) or a

pint of beer comes to around 230 calories, which is similar to eating a small bar of chocolate or an ice cream.

Q & A

What if I'm not losing weight?

When you switch to the New 5:2 you should continue to lose weight at a rate of 2.2–4.4 lb a week. If this doesn't happen straightaway, be patient. If it really doesn't happen and you still have weight to lose, then I would suggest you look seriously at what you are eating on your nonfast days. Take photos. Keep a record. Include absolutely everything. Come and talk to people on the website.

The alternative, of course, is that you increase your number of 800-calorie days: a friend of mine started on 5:2, found he wasn't losing weight as fast as he wanted, so he moved on to 2:5, eating his 800 calories across the week, then having a bit of a splurge at the weekend. Or you could go back to the Very Fast800 for a while, just to kick-start your system.

Is it safe to fast on my period?

You shouldn't be fasting if you are pregnant or breast-feeding. But there is no reason why you shouldn't do 800-calorie days while on your period, unless your periods are particularly heavy or painful. If this is the case, it is worth having your iron levels tested and taking a supplement if they are low.

Will fasting affect my sleep?

Some people struggle with hunger, particularly during the first two weeks, and that can disturb your sleep. I found that adding in TRE improved my sleep. Why? Dr. Panda thinks this may be because shortly before you fall asleep your core temperature starts to fall. It is a cue to your brain that it is time for a bit of shut-eye. If your body is still trying to digest food when you go to bed (and digesting a big meal can take many hours), this will not happen.

What about exercise?

As with the Very Fast800, you should stick with your existing regimen, and try to add in some of the exercises that I recommended in Chapter 5. Being active is a great way of distracting yourself and will boost your mood.

There is increasing evidence that exercising in tandem with TRE can enhance its effectiveness. TRE is popular with athletes and body builders because they find that it enables them to lose fat but preserve muscle. In a recent randomized study[35] of fit young men, those put on a 16:8 diet for eight weeks lost significant amounts of fat but remained as muscled, and as strong, as a control group who were not fasting. This could be because not eating for 16 hours a day gives the body time to repair the mitochondria, the tiny structures that act like batteries to power our muscles. An extended overnight fast also ensures that old, damaged muscle cells are broken down and replaced with new ones.

STAGE 3: KEEPING THE WEIGHT OFF AS A WAY OF LIFE

Once you have hit your targets, celebrate. Tell your friends. You have done something that is really tough and you don't want to go back to your old ways. If you have followed this program you will already have made changes that will set you up for long-term success:

1. *You will be feeling better,* with more energy—happier, brighter and lighter, even more confident and back in control.

2. *You will have lost a lot of weight, fast.* Large and rapid weight loss, as I've said already, is a great predictor of long-term success.

3. *You will have preserved your muscle mass and therefore your metabolic rate* by doing a low-carb, Mediterranean diet and maintaining an exercise regimen.

4. *Having embraced the low-carb Mediterranean-style diet,* you can now fit in some "treat days," but go carefully. Occasional lapses are fine, but if you return to your old ways, you will return to your old prediet body.

5. *You have managed the New 5:2,* so there is no reason why you shouldn't stick to doing 5:2 or 6:1 long term. Doing the 6:1 (where you fast one day a week) is an excellent option for keeping your body in good shape, particularly if you are happy with your current weight and haven't found intermittent fasting too stressful.

6. *You will hopefully have found that TRE suits you,* and if you want to continue, long term, there is no reason why you shouldn't just keep going. Most people find 10:14 or 12:12 is doable, albeit with occasional lapses. If you find yourself having a late-night meal/snack/drink, then aim for a later breakfast.

7. *You have gained future health benefits, which is very motivating.* By losing visceral fat and changing what you eat, you will have reduced your risk of many chronic diseases. People with high blood pressure report significant improvements. Many people with type 2 diabetes or prediabetes tell me

their blood sugar levels have returned to normal, without medication. People with a fatty liver should have seen their liver health transformed (rapid weight loss is currently the only effective treatment for nonalcoholic fatty liver disease, also known as NAFLD). Intermittent fasting has been shown to reduce inflammation, improving conditions such as arthritis, eczema, psoriasis, and asthma. And hopefully your cholesterol profile will be looking better too.

8. *You have embraced a new way of life—for life.*
   For many people, simply sticking to a relatively low-carb, Med-style diet, while managing portion control is enough. And if things slip, you know exactly what to do . . .

So what else can you do to ensure long-term success? There's no doubt that over the next few months you will face challenges, whether at home or at work, but try not to let these knock you off course. The longer you keep the weight off, the easier it will become.

This is a list of some of the most successful strategies that I, and others, have adopted to stay on track:

- **Keep junk food out of the house.** This is the number one strategy used by successful dieters. However strong-willed you are, however long it has been since you ate a tub of ice cream on your own, there is always the risk that if the food is close at hand you will eat it. A distinguished surgeon recently told me he did the FastDiet and lost 56 lb after being called a "fat bastard" by a fellow surgeon. Now he's lost all that weight, he has a number of simple rules that keep him slim. These include never keeping sugary treats in the house and only eating ice cream when he goes to the movies. Since he hardly ever goes to the movies this is not a problem.

- **Weigh yourself regularly.** Surprisingly enough, lots of studies have shown that regular self-weighing is one of the best ways to maintain weight loss. Daily is better than weekly, and weekly is better than monthly. A recent large study[36] of over 1,700 people followed for more than two years found that those who weighed themselves daily were, on average, 14.3 lb lighter at the end of the trial than those who weighed themselves monthly. I weigh myself most days first thing in the morning, soon after I get up. I know that my weight can fluctuate, depending on how dehydrated I am, but if my weight starts to creep up I respond.

- **Buy yourself a set of new clothes when you finish the diet.** You deserve a reward for all your hard work, but a new wardrobe will also help keep you on your toes. Dave, who lost over 44 lb in

12 weeks and reversed his diabetes, now has a favorite shirt that he uses as a measure of how well he is sticking to his new habits. He told me that when the shirt starts getting tight, he knows it is time to do a bit more fasting.

- **If you do start to put on weight you must take action as quickly as possible.** A weight gain of more than a few pounds is likely to lead to despair and extensive weight regain. Instead of blaming yourself, act. Go back on to 800 calories. Use those meal replacement shakes that are still in the cupboard. Knock the weight regain on the head before it really sets in.
- **Keep active.** Along with regular self-weighing, increased activity is something that most successful long-term dieters mention. The good news is that when people lose weight they find that activities like walking or cycling become easier and much more enjoyable.
- **Self-monitoring.** If one of the reasons you decided to go on the diet was because your blood sugars were too high, then regular self-testing with a finger-prick monitor is a useful thing to do. Many people, having reversed their type 2 diabetes by rapid weight loss, use the fear of developing type 2 diabetes again as a powerful motivator. I keep a close eye on my blood sugar levels and my blood pressure, as well as my weight.

- **Join an online community and share your data.** A study by Northwestern University[37] found that online dieters with high "social embeddedness"— the ones who logged on regularly, recorded their weigh-ins, and "friended" other members— were those who lost the most weight and kept it off, long term. As one of the researchers on the study, Dr. Louis Amaral, pointed out, "If you monitor your weight, you are engaged. If you communicate online with other people you are even more engaged. And when you need support you will get it."

- **If your friends, colleagues, or your partner are overweight or obese**, try to persuade them to give this diet a go. We are social creatures and we tend to mimic the people around us. One study[38] found that when people lose weight with a partner they are far more likely to keep it off than when they do it alone. Your partner can be your greatest ally (mine is), or they can sometimes undermine your efforts. If your partner isn't supportive, then it is even more important that you find friends or an online community to help you through the hard times.

- **Always try to sit down for meals and never eat on the move.** This counts whether you are getting something out of the fridge, cooking the kids' snack, clearing up their plates, walking around a supermarket, or being offered a piece of obscure posh cheese. All of these grazing moments add up, and not in a good way.

- **Find healthy foods to eat during the day** at work, and when out and about—and don't be embarrassed to prepare something in advance. Packed lunches are going to be healthier than something from a snack bar, and will save you money.

- **Put less food on your plate than you think you might actually eat** and only help yourself to seconds after a pause, if you're still hungry. If you do want more, try to make it mainly nonstarchy vegetables. It takes time for the food you eat to get to the receptors in your small intestine that signal "enough," so the faster you eat, the more you eat. Piling up your plate will encourage you to overeat.

- **Be mindful.** I wrote about mindfulness in the previous chapter and about different ways you can remain "mindful" throughout the day. A recent analysis of 19 studies[39] found that mindfulness-based interventions increased weight loss and reduced "obesity-related eating behaviors." Do give it a go.

- **Write things down.** A study by Kaiser Permanente's Center for Health Research,[40] one of the largest and longest weight-loss maintenance trials ever conducted, found that those who kept daily food records lost twice as much weight as those who didn't. It seems that the simple act of writing down what you eat encourages people to consume fewer calories. It doesn't have to be that complicated. Just scribble it down in a notebook or on your cell phone. Send yourself emails tallying each meal, or send yourself a text message. It is the process of reflecting on what you are eating that makes you aware of the bad habits you might be slipping into.

- **Prioritize sleep.** Most people need at least seven to eight hours sleep a night, and if you try to get by on less than that you are likely to experience increased hunger and cravings, particularly for high-carb, high-calorie foods. Getting a good night's sleep is all about establishing a regular schedule, in which you go to bed and get up at much the same time every day, whether it is during the week or the weekend. Too little sleep will increase your stress hormones, making you hungrier and more likely to overeat, which in turn will make you sleep less. It's a vicious cycle.

- **Above all, remind yourself why you are doing this.** I want to live to a healthy old age, enjoying life with friends and family. That's why keeping my weight down is so important to me. Whatever your motives, remind yourself of them from time to time. Revisit you original goals. Losing weight and keeping it off is one of the hardest things I've done. But I've succeeded and so can you. And as with adopting any new habit—it really does get easier with time. Good luck and let us know how you get on at thefast800.com.

8

SUPERSIZE ME

As I mentioned in the introduction, when I was researching this book—and following my own personal rationale that I should try the programs I recommend—I tested out the Fast800, by putting on weight and then seeing how quickly I could lose it again.

Before starting, I did a range of tests, including measuring my fasting glucose, my blood pressure, my weight, and my waist.

The tests showed I was basically healthy. I came in at 172 lb, with a waist of 32 inches, blood sugars and blood pressure both excellent. Time to undo all that.

To put on weight, I stuck to a relatively healthy diet but increased my consumption of starches. I ate more bread, potatoes, rice, and pasta, plus the occasional cookie.

Here's an entry from my diary: "It's now a couple of weeks since I started doing my experiment and the biggest surprise has been that, so far, I have put on remarkably little weight. I think my body has just gotten used to my current weight and is resisting my attempt to pile on the fat. In some ways that is immensely reassuring. I could get used to this new lifestyle."

It didn't last.

"It's now a month into my experiment and the scales are beginning to move. My blood sugar levels are also starting to rise. The strangest and most unsettling thing is that I am now really beginning to crave sweet things again. I find it almost impossible to pass a shop and not buy a small bar of chocolate. Clare says that I am beginning to snore again and she is anxious that I stop soon."

In the end, it took me nearly four months to put on 14 lb and by then the rot had really set in. My blood sugars were almost back in the diabetic range. My waist had ballooned to 37 inches and my blood pressure was the red zone. I felt hungry much of the time.

I was doing a lot of filming during that period and I worried that people would notice that I'd put on lots of weight and ask why I had allowed myself to go to seed, but no one did. It helps that when I put on fat it is mainly internal. Wearing baggy shirts also helps.

My wife told me I was beginning to look older. I was sleeping badly and feeling increasingly moody.

So, after a final, indulgent summer vacation in Greece, I knuckled down to losing weight. I started by doing the Very Fast800 program, sticking to 800 calories a day, and using menus from this book.

I included TRE, doing a 12:12 program. My plan was to finish eating by 8 p.m. and then not eat anything till at least 8 a.m. the next morning.

So how did I get on?

Well, it was easier than I feared. Perhaps because I am used to occasional fasting, sticking to 800 calories a day was not as challenging as I thought it would be. I knew what to expect, which helps, and I imagine that my body is more used to "flipping the metabolic switch." I was certainly hungry and a bit grumpy to begin with, but after a few days the cravings and the bursts of hungriness passed. Mostly.

Since I was trying to fit this rapid weight-loss diet around a busy filming schedule, I had to combine using meal replacement shakes when I was on the road with recipes from this book when I was at home. On a couple of occasions I had to go for business-related meals, but I managed to stick to fish and vegetables.

The weight loss was fast and the metabolic changes impressive. In the first four days I lost 6 lb, some of it water. My blood sugars and my blood pressure also fell. Optimistically, I tried to tighten my belt by a notch. Not there yet.

I kept up my exercise regimen, but I did notice that going for long walks or runs was tougher than it had been. Although I was in mild ketosis (I used my ketone sticks to check), my energy levels were definitely lower.

I was glugging back lots of water and black tea, so neither headaches nor constipation were a problem.

I had some bad moments, including one occasion when I was stranded on a railway platform at 10 p.m., not having eaten that day, with nothing for company but a chocolate machine. Fortunately I didn't have any change, or I would probably have cracked.

There were lapses. There was an evening when I gave myself a night off and drank several glasses of wine, followed by way too much cheese. And another occasion when I gave in to one slice of hot buttered toast, then another. But on the whole I stayed on track.

After two weeks I had managed to lose 11 lb and get my blood sugars and blood pressure back to normal. I could have continued on the rapid weight-loss program but I thought this would be a good moment to switch to the 5:2.

As an experiment, I did my fast days back-to-back (Mondays and Tuesdays) and noticed, thanks to my keto measuring sticks, that I was in mild ketosis for some of the first and most of the second day.

Doing exercise became easier. I could push myself harder without feeling drained.

I continued to eat the Med-style menus from the book on my fast days and eat more freely on the nonfast days. I also returned to drinking wine on my nonfast days. It was, dare I say it, easy.

Three weeks and five days after I started, I was back

to my previous healthy weight and everything else had returned to normal.

What had I learned?

- That this diet is very doable.
- That if I let myself go, then the diabetes and other health issues will return.
- That what I eat really does affect my mood.
- That TRE helps, but it is tricky to stick to rigidly if you have a social life. That said, I will persist with trying to do it on as many occasions as possible, as I think the science is convincing.

Where do we go from here?

It is six years since I first suggested that intermittent fasting might offer a new and exciting alternative to the standard "slow, steady, eat low-fat" message. Today I am more confident than ever that it does.

I am stopped on the streets almost every day by people who want to tell me about their weight-loss success. Do I mind? Not at all. I love feedback and even if we never cross paths you can always get in contact with me or the Fast800 team via the website.

Just as important, I feel that the science is coming along in leaps and bounds. Although there are still some very important questions that remain unresolved, answers are on their way.

So will Professor Valter Longo's Fast Mimicking Diet turn out to be as revolutionary as his early studies suggest it might be?

Will Professor Mark Mattson's 5:2 study on the brain open the door to a new way of combating dementia?

Will doctors and other health professionals respond positively to the latest research showing just how effective a rapid weight-loss diet can be?

I'm obviously hoping the answers to all these questions will be "yes."

Intermittent fasting has changed my life. I hope it changes yours.

RECIPES

by Dr. Clare Bailey

and nutritional therapist Joy Skipper

This section contains lots of ideas for how to make up your 800 calories on fast days—whether you want to have three small meals or two larger ones. There are also options for making a dish a bit "more substantial" with minimal added calories, and for making larger portions for nonfast days. All calorie counts are per portion.

BREAKFAST

These easy suggestions for filling breakfasts will neither significantly increase your blood sugars, nor lead to weight gain. And because they keep you full for longer, you are less likely to be overcome by the urge to snack.

It's fine if you don't eat breakfast—in fact, it extends your fasting window; but it is important to increase your fluid intake if you skip a meal, or are on an 800-calorie day (see page 252 for drink suggestions). Some of the recipes are portable, so you can take them with you and eat them later in the morning, or even for lunch.

Boiled Eggs with Spiced Asparagus Soldiers
230 calories
Serves 2

A fabulous light breakfast that is full of flavor.

8 oz asparagus spears
4 large eggs
½ tbsp olive oil
Large pinch of ground cumin or smoked paprika

1. Cut or break off the woody ends of the asparagus and blanch the spears in a pan of boiling water for 3 minutes. Drain them and set aside.
2. Heat a pan of water to a rolling boil. Add the eggs and cook for 6–7 minutes for a soft yolk.
3. Meanwhile, heat a grill pan on the stove top. In a medium bowl, toss the asparagus spears in the oil and sprinkle them with the cumin and some salt and freshly ground black pepper. Cook for 3–4 minutes, turning them a few times, until they are tender and slightly charred.
4. Serve the eggs in egg cups or ramekins, with the asparagus for dunking!

MORE SUBSTANTIAL (Additions show calories per portion): Add a large handful of spinach, tossed for 1–2 minutes in a nonstick pan until it wilts (insignificant calories; add 37 calories if you use 1 tsp butter, or 27 calories for 1 tsp olive oil).

Baked Eggs 2 Ways

These "muffins" taste equally delicious hot from the oven or popped in a lunchbox to eat later.

Easy Bacon and Egg Muffins
280 calories
Serves 2

4 bacon strips
4 large eggs
1 tsp grated Parmesan

1. Preheat the oven to 400°F. Lightly grease 4 holes of a metal or silicone muffin tray. Or use ovenproof ramekins, lightly greased.
2. Cut the bacon strips in half and lay them, crisscrossed, in the muffin holes.
3. Crack 1 egg into each hole.
4. Sprinkle the Parmesan on top, along with some freshly ground black pepper. Bake for 15 minutes for a soft yolk, or 20 minutes for a hard yolk.

MORE OPTIONS: Add 2–3 tbsp sliced cooked greens (such as spinach, kale, Swiss chard) or 3 large cremini mushrooms, diced and dry-fried in a nonstick pan (insignificant calories), or fried in ½ tbsp olive oil (add 30 calories per person).

Baked Salmon and Eggs with Chives
300 calories
Serves 2

Salmon provides a healthy omega-3 boost for your brain and circulation, and helps reduce inflammation.

5–6 oz smoked salmon
Handful of fresh baby spinach or leftover greens, chopped
4 large eggs
1 tbsp chives, chopped (optional)
2 tsp grated Parmesan

1. Preheat the oven to 400°F. Lightly grease 4 holes of a metal or silicone muffin tray. Alternatively, use ovenproof ramekins, lightly greased.
2. Line the 4 holes with the smoked salmon.
3. Place the spinach in a bowl. Using a fork, lightly whisk in the eggs, chives, and some freshly ground black pepper.
4. Divide the mixture among the 4 holes. Sprinkle with the Parmesan and some more black pepper and bake for 15 minutes, or until the eggs look set.

MORE SUBSTANTIAL: Serve them with extra leafy greens such as arugula or baby salad leaves on the side (insignificant calories).

Porridge with Pistachios and Chia
370 calories
Serves 2

Creamy porridge with a hint of exotic cardamom, and the added benefit of chia, a superfood high in nutrients, fiber, and protein.

¼ cup rolled oats
1¼ cups milk
1 tbsp chia seeds
½ tsp cardamom seeds
Handful of chopped pistachios

Place all the ingredients in a pan and bring to a boil. Reduce the heat and simmer for 6–8 minutes, stirring occasionally, until the porridge is thick and creamy.

MORE SUBSTANTIAL: Serve it topped with a handful of raspberries, blueberries, or the pulp of a passion fruit (add 15 calories for 1½ oz).

Speedy Eggs and Avocado
290 calories
Serves 1

This is one for people who say they don't have time to cook eggs for breakfast—prepare them the day before, then assemble the dish in the morning.

2 large eggs
½ medium avocado
Squeeze of lemon

1. Cook the eggs for 6–7 minutes in a pan of boiling water, then place them under cold running water. Peel them and put them in the fridge (if you're preparing them in advance).
2. In the morning, pit, peel, and slice the avocado. Place it on a plate and squeeze the lemon juice over it.
3. Cut the eggs into quarters. Mix them with the avocado slices and some seasoning.

MORE SUBSTANTIAL: Serve the mixture on a slice of rye bread (add 55 calories) or whole wheat sourdough toast (add 72 calories).

Tomato and Basil Omelet

240 calories
Serves 1

Get the day off to a healthy start with this classic Mediterranean-style omelet.

2 large eggs
½ tbsp olive oil
3 cherry tomatoes, halved
4–5 basil leaves, shredded

1. Beat the eggs in a bowl with a fork. Add a little seasoning.
2. Heat the oil in a small frying pan and cook the cherry tomatoes for 2 minutes.
3. Add the basil, cook for another 20 seconds, then pour in the eggs, swirling them around the pan with a wooden spatula.
4. Once the omelet starts to set, loosen the edges and fold it over. When it is lightly golden, slide it onto a warm plate to serve.

MORE SUBSTANTIAL: Serve it with a large handful of baby salad leaves or arugula (insignificant calories, unless you use a dressing, such as the olive oil and apple cider vinegar dressing on page 244—add 100 calories).

Creamy Green Smoothie
165 calories
Serves 2

½ cucumber, chopped
2 celery stalks, chopped
1 kiwi fruit, chopped
1 large egg
2 tbsp extra-virgin olive oil

Blitz all the ingredients together in a blender with some seasoning and ⅔ cup water. Pour it into 2 glasses and serve immediately.

Spiced Mango Smoothie
190 calories
Serves 2

1 large mango, peeled, pitted, and cut into chunks
1 tbsp full-fat Greek yogurt
1¼ cups almond milk
Zest and juice of ½ orange
¾-inch piece fresh ginger, peeled and grated
¼ tsp ground cinnamon, plus extra to serve
Large pinch of ground turmeric

Blitz all the ingredients together in a blender. Pour it into 2 glasses and serve with some ground cinnamon sprinkled on top.

LIGHT MEALS

In an ideal world, following the traditional "Mediterranean" way of eating, we would all eat our main meal early in the day, because that way it is less likely to be stored as fat. However, clearly, this doesn't work for everyone, and so in this section dishes have been divided into "light" and "main" meals, rather than "lunch" or "dinner," so you can be flexible about when you eat them.

The light meals are generally simple and quick to make, and usually lower in calories than the mains. Some work well as a brunch.

Our recommendation is that you don't snack between meals, as this stops fat burning.

Hummus in a Hurry
205 calories
Makes 4 portions

An almost instant meal which fills the gap and tastes great served with some crunchy vegetables. Don't worry about the generous amount of olive oil—it adds to both the taste and the health benefits.

7 oz canned chickpeas
2 tbsp lemon juice, or more to taste
2½ tbsp extra-virgin olive oil
½ tbsp tahini
2 garlic cloves, chopped

1. Drain the chickpeas, reserving the liquid.
2. Blend all the ingredients together, except for ½ tbsp oil.
3. Add a little of the reserved chickpea liquid if needed to get the desired consistency. Season the hummus with salt and freshly ground black pepper to taste.
4. Drizzle the remaining oil on top, along with some cumin seeds or paprika, if you wish. Serve with crispy vegetable crudités, such as sticks of celery, cucumber and zucchini, baby asparagus, and cauliflower or broccoli florets, all of which contain very few calories and are a good source of fiber, so can be eaten almost freely.

TIP: Don't over-squeeze the lemon when you juice it, as the white pith can make the juice bitter.

Tapenade with Feta
138 calories
Serves 2

Olive paste can have an overwhelmingly intense and sharp taste, but combined here with feta, it makes a delicately tangy, creamy spread. Delicious on coin-shaped slices of zucchini as canapés, or spread on seeded crackers—or simply served as a dip.

1½ oz feta cheese
1½ oz pitted olives, from a jar or can, drained
1 tbsp olive oil

Blitz the ingredients together with a handheld blender in a small bowl, leaving some chunky bits of olive.

NONFAST DAYS: Just eat more of it!

Crunchy Zucchini Canapés 3 Ways

The new blini. So easy and so healthy too. You don't have to count the calories in the zucchini, as they are so low as to be insignificant. Top the slices with flavored cream cheese, pickled fish, chives, Quick Pickled Fennel and Radishes (page 237) or whatever healthy leftovers you can assemble from the fridge. Finish them off with a spoonful of home-made sauerkraut or kimchi (see pages 240–41).

½ medium zucchini, sliced approx. ¼ inch thick

Toppings:
- 1 tbsp Tapenade with Feta (page 180)
  62 calories
- 1 tbsp Hummus in a Hurry (page 179)
  46 calories
- 1 tbsp Smashed Avocado (page 182)
  103 calories

Dark Rye Bread 2 Ways:

Most breads, including many "brown" varieties, are made with highly processed flour, from which the majority of the beneficial nutrients and fiber have been removed. Although "brown" bread may contain healthy whole grains or seeds, these are often token in quantity. Whole grain dark rye is usually higher in fiber. If you find the taste of dark rye bread too strong, look for the lighter versions. Alternatively, use seeded whole wheat or brown sourdough bread.

Smashed Avocado on Dark Rye Bread
290 calories
Serves 2

1 large avocado, pitted and peeled
Juice of ½ small lemon
1 tbsp extra-virgin olive oil
2 thin slices rye bread
2 tbsp pumpkin or sunflower seeds, toasted

1. Coarsely mash the avocado in a bowl with the lemon juice and oil, leaving some chunky bits.
2. Season it with salt and freshly ground black pepper and spoon it onto the slices of rye bread.
3. Sprinkle the toasted seeds over the top before serving.

Dark Rye Bread with Egg and Spinach
240 calories
Serves 1

2 large eggs
1 tsp butter or olive oil
2 handfuls of spinach
1 slice of rye bread, toasted

1. Either poach the eggs in boiling water for
   4 minutes or scramble them.
2. Meanwhile, melt the butter or oil in a nonstick
   frying pan over medium heat and add the spinach.
   Cook briefly, until the spinach just wilts, then
   spoon it onto the toast.
3. Place the eggs on top. Season to taste with a little
   salt and plenty of freshly ground black pepper.

TIP: For extra flavor add a few drops of Tabasco sauce or a
pinch of cayenne pepper.

Turmeric Spiced Mushroom Omelet
210 calories
Serves 1

Enjoy this lightly spiced, superhealthy omelet for breakfast, lunch, or supper.

1 tsp coconut oil or butter
2 cremini mushrooms, diced
1 green onion, diced
½ tsp ground turmeric
¼ tsp red pepper flakes, or to taste
2 large eggs, lightly whisked
Small handful of fresh cilantro, chopped

1. Place the oil in a small frying pan over medium heat and cook the mushrooms and green onion for 3–4 minutes.
2. Stir in the turmeric and red pepper flakes, then after another minute, pour in the eggs along with some seasoning.
3. Stir the eggs lightly and cook gently for a few minutes, until they begin to set but are still slightly soft and runny on the surface.
4. Scatter the cilantro on top, then fold the omelet in half and slide it onto a plate.

TIP: Michael loves to eat this omelet with 1 tbsp fermented cabbage to add some contrasting tang and crunch (see page 240). If you are even more adventurous, try topping it with ½ tbsp kimchi, for a tsunami of exotic flavor.

MORE SUBSTANTIAL: Serve the omelet with half a plateful of steamed greens or colored leafy vegetables (no calorie counting needed) or salad leaves (add calories if you use a dressing, such as olive oil and apple cider vinegar dressing, see page 244).

Sliced Ham or Halloumi with Purple Slaw
200 calories
Serves 2

This versatile crunchy slaw goes well with any cold meat or cheese. If made in advance, it makes an easy, almost instant lunch that is packed with protein, fiber, and healthy fats.

For the slaw:
¼ small red cabbage, finely sliced (about 6 oz), see Tips
¼ small green cabbage, finely sliced (about 6 oz),
   see Tips
1 green onion, finely sliced
4 oz cooked ham, or 2 oz halloumi (see Tips)

For the dressing:
2 tbsp full-fat Greek yogurt
1 tsp Dijon mustard
1 tbsp extra-virgin olive oil

1. To make the dressing, whisk all the ingredients together with some seasoning.
2. Mix the sliced cabbage and green onion in a bowl.
3. Add the yogurt dressing and mix everything together well.
4. Serve the slaw with the ham.

TIPS: If using halloumi, slice it and fry it with a tiny drizzle of olive oil in a nonstick frying pan until it is golden on both sides. If cooking for one, the second portion of slaw will keep for a day or two. If you don't have both red and white cabbage, just double the quantity of the one you have.

MORE SUBSTANTIAL: Serve it with a pile of green and colored leaves and fresh herbs (no calorie counting required). Vegetarians can increase the protein by adding 2 tbsp nutritional yeast and an extra spoonful of yogurt to the dressing.

NONFAST DAYS: Serve it with an extra slice of ham. You could also add half a packet (4½ oz) of cooked puy lentils per person for extra protein or 2–3 heaping tbsp cooked brown rice or quinoa.

Lemon and Thyme Chicken Kebabs
220 calories
Serves 2

Not only do chicken thighs contain more nutrients than breast meat, they are also more succulent and flavorful. Kebabs are well designed for eating on the hoof—take them to work in a lunchbox with a generous salad and a dressing in a small jar.

4 boneless, skinless chicken thighs, diced
   (about 8 oz)
Juice and zest of ½ lemon
½ tsp dried thyme
1 garlic clove, crushed
1 tbsp olive oil
1 medium onion, cut into 8 pieces

1. Mix the chicken in a bowl with the lemon, thyme, garlic, and oil and season well with salt and freshly ground black pepper. Let marinate for 2 hours, if time permits.
2. Heat the broiler to maximum. Divide the chicken and onion pieces among 4 skewers.
3. Place the skewers on a grill pan under the broiler for about 15 minutes, turning them frequently, until the chicken is cooked through and golden brown.

TIP: If using wooden skewers remember to soak them in water for 10 minutes before broiling so they don't burn.

MORE SUBSTANTIAL: Serve the kebabs with a handful of green and colored leafy salad (no calorie counting required). Add a dressing such as the olive oil and apple cider vinegar on page 244 (add 100 calories).

NONFAST DAY: Double the portion and add 2–3 tbsp cooked brown rice.

Minced Pork and Snow Pea Stir-Fry with Noodles
320 calories
Serves 2

Fast comfort food—hot, filling, and bursting with flavor.

7 oz ground pork
1½ tbsp soy sauce
1 tsp cornstarch
1¼ cups chicken or vegetable stock (½ stock cube)
4 oz Zero noodles, rinsed, or soba noodles (see Tips)
1½ tbsp coconut or rapeseed oil
¾-inch piece fresh ginger, peeled and diced
1 onion, chopped
7 oz snow peas or thin green beans

1. Place the pork in a nonmetallic bowl with ½ tbsp soy sauce, a generous amount of freshly ground black pepper, and the cornstarch. Mix everything together well and marinate for 30 minutes if you have time.
2. Add the remaining soy sauce to the stock in a pitcher.
3. Cook the noodles according to the package instructions, then drain and rinse them under cold water.
4. Place a wok over high heat until it starts to smoke. Add the oil and stir-fry the pork for 3–4 minutes, or until it is lightly browned.
5. Reduce the heat to medium and toss in the ginger

and onion. Stir-fry for a few more minutes, then add the snow peas. After another minute, pour in the stock and the noodles and bring the wok back to a simmer, stirring frequently, for 1 minute.

TIPS: Serve the stir-fry sprinkled with ½–1 tsp red pepper flakes if you like a bit of extra heat. You can easily substitute Quorn for the pork. Zero noodles are made of konjac, a plant-based complex carbohydrate that provides gut-friendly fiber while releasing very little starchy carbohydrate (available in big supermarkets and online). If using soba noodles, cook them al dente and rinse them in cold water before use (add 176 calories).

NONFAST DAY: Use a medium portion of whole wheat noodles or soba noodles and add 1 tsp sesame oil along with some extra sliced crispy vegetables at step 5.

Instant Miso Soup with Mushrooms and Greens
23 calories
Serves 1

A simple miso soup that is very low in calories, yet surprisingly satisfying. Take the ingredients to work in a jar—and simply top up with boiling water.

1 miso soup sachet
1 medium mushroom, finely sliced
Small handful of baby spinach or cooked greens, shredded
A few sprigs of fresh parsley or cilantro (optional)

1. Pour the contents of the miso packet into a good-sized bowl or mug.
2. Stir in 1 cup boiling water, then add the mushroom and the greens. Let sit for 3–5 minutes to allow the mushroom to soften.

MORE SUBSTANTIAL: Add 1 tbsp heated diced cooked chicken or some shrimp or tofu (see Extras on pages 243–45 for other options to add).

WHAT DOES AN 800-CALORIE DAY LOOK LIKE?

Spiced Mango Smoothie 190 calories (page 177)
Minced Pork and Snow Peas Stir-Fry with Noodles 320 calories (page 190)
Haddock Steamed with Thai Spices 300 calories (page 226)

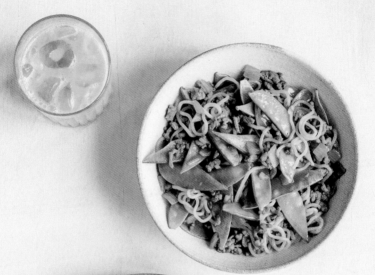

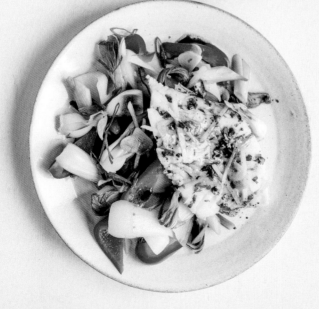

Boiled Eggs with Spiced Asparagus Soldiers 230 calories (page 171)
Root Vegetables and Turmeric Soup 170 calories (page 194)
Spanish Eggplant Stew with Chorizo 390 calories (page 213)

Speedy Eggs and Avocado 290 calories (page 175)
Miso Eggplant "Steaks" with Roasted Carrots and Cashews 315 calories (page 202)
Lemon and Thyme Chicken Kebabs 220 calories (page 188)

Baked Salmon and Eggs with Chives 300 calories (page 173)
Crunchy Zucchini Canapés 3 Ways 211 calories (page 181)
Garlic Shrimp with Mixed Zucchini Noodles and Spaghetti 290 calories
(page 198)

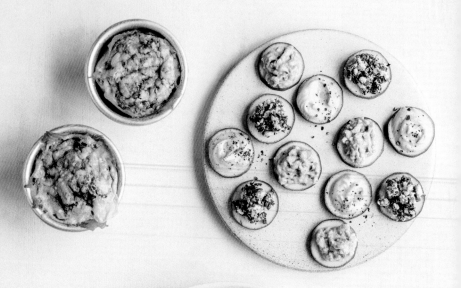

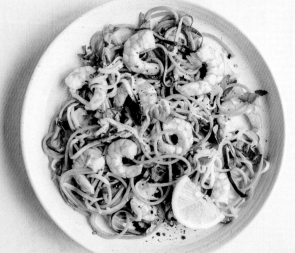

Smashed Avocado on Dark Rye Bread 290 calories (page 182)
Sausage and Mushrooms with Spring Greens 545 calories (page 219)

Pearl Barley and Pumpkin Seed Salad 340 calories (page 208)
Peppered Roast Cod with Nutty Broccoli 430 calories (page 224)

Porridge with Pistachios and Chia 370 calories (page 174)
Speedy Chinese Salmon Stir-Fry 360 calories (page 210)

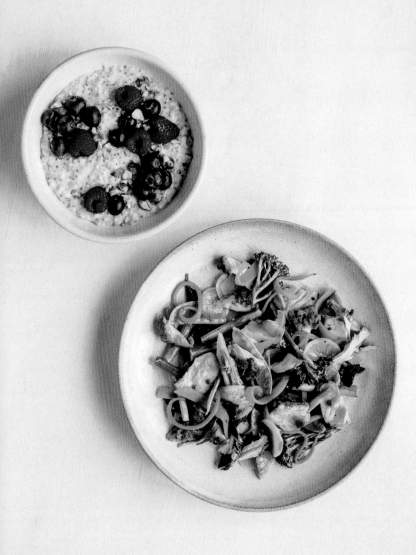

Pasta and Pesto Salad Jar 495 calories (page 207)
Shrimp Korma with Coconut Cauli Rice 320 calories (page 228)

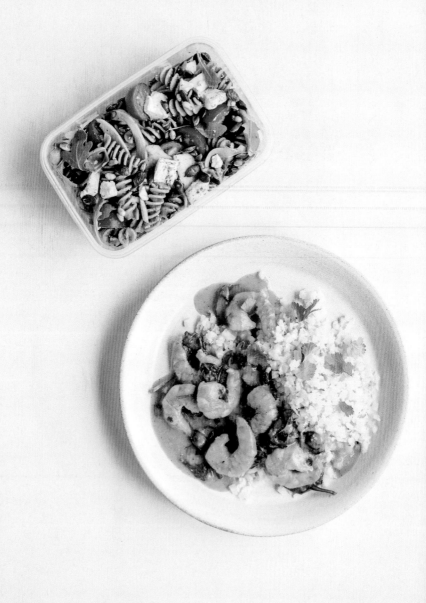

Quick 'n' Easy Pea and Spinach Soup
130 calories
Serves 2

A glorious green and filling soup to keep you going during the day.

8 oz frozen peas
4 oz frozen spinach
1 garlic clove, chopped
½ chicken or vegetable bouillon cube
2 tbsp full-fat Greek yogurt

1. Place all the ingredients except the yogurt in a medium saucepan over medium heat. Add 2 cups water and bring it to a boil.
2. Season the soup generously with freshly ground black pepper, and allow it to simmer for about 5 minutes. Then remove it from the heat and blitz it with a handheld blender or in a food processor, leaving some texture.
3. Share the soup between 2 bowls and dollop 1 tbsp of yogurt in each.

MORE SUBSTANTIAL: Add another tbsp yogurt to each bowl (37 calories) or drizzle over ½ tbsp olive oil (49 calories).

NONFAST DAY: Add yogurt or olive oil as above. Eat with a slice of whole grain sourdough bread.

Root Vegetables and Turmeric Soup
170 calories
Serves 4

For this comforting soup, the root vegetables are cooked with their skins on to retain all their excellent nutrients. The turmeric gives an extra health boost, with its well-proven anti-inflammatory properties, which are enhanced by the addition of black pepper.

3 tbsp olive oil
1 onion, peeled and diced
1 tsp ground cumin
2 tsp ground turmeric
14 oz celeriac, scrubbed and chopped
12 oz parsnips, scrubbed and chopped
5¼ cups vegetable or chicken stock

1. Heat the oil in a large pan and sauté the onion until it is soft but not browned. Add the spices, and after about 1 minute, stir in the vegetables.
2. Pour in the stock and bring it to a boil. Cover the pan and simmer for about 20 minutes, or until the vegetables are soft.
3. Remove the pan from the heat and blend the soup with a handheld blender until smooth.
4. Season it to taste with salt and freshly ground black pepper.

TIP: For added flavor, scatter a handful of chopped parsley or cilantro, or a pinch of red pepper flakes on top.

Red Lentil and Coconut Soup

280 calories
Serves 4

A tasty, aromatic soup packed with fiber and protein.

3 tsp coriander seeds, lightly crushed
2 tsp cumin seeds
1 tbsp olive oil
2 leeks, trimmed and thinly sliced
3 garlic cloves, crushed
⅔ cup red lentils
1½ cups canned light coconut milk
Juice of ½ lime
2½ cups vegetable stock
2 tbsp flaked almonds, toasted

1. Toast the coriander and cumin seeds in a large saucepan over low heat for 2–3 minutes, until they become fragrant. Remove them from the pan.
2. Heat the oil in the same pan and sauté the leeks and garlic with plenty of freshly ground black pepper for 4–5 minutes.
3. Stir in the seeds and lentils and cook for 1 minute before pouring in the coconut milk, lime juice, and stock. Add a pinch of salt and bring the pan to a boil. Then reduce the heat and simmer for 25 minutes, or until the lentils are tender.
4. Serve the soup in warmed bowls, sprinkled with the flaked almonds.

NONFAST DAY: Add a small piece of whole grain pita.

Gut-Healing Chicken Broth
Makes about 8 cups

A popular dish from *The Clever Gut Cookbook*, this nourishing broth contains very few calories and will keep you going on an 800-calorie day. Slow-cooking releases the minerals and nutrients from the bones.

3 tbsp olive oil
4 celery stalks, coarsely chopped
2 small onions, chopped
2 leeks, trimmed
1 large garlic clove, halved
2 carrots, chopped
2 lb pasture-raised chicken wings and/or
    chicken carcasses
1 tbsp apple cider vinegar
2 bay leaves
1 bouquet garni
Handful of parsley sprigs
6–8 black peppercorns

1. Heat the oil in a large pan with a lid and sauté the celery, onions, and leeks for 5–7 minutes.
2. Add the garlic, carrots, chicken, vinegar, bay leaves, and bouquet garni.
3. Add 8 cups water and bring to a simmer. Cover and cook for 3–4 hours, or ideally for 5–6 hours, to extract all the nutrients from the bones. Check occasionally that it has not dried out and top up with water, if needed, skimming any gray scum from the surface.

196

4. Pour the stock through a sieve into a bowl and
   allow it to drain for 15 minutes. For a thicker,
   tastier broth, gently press the soft vegetables
   through the sieve with a spoon.
5. Serve the soup immediately or let it cool, then ladle
   it into containers to store in the fridge for up to
   5 days, or in the freezer.

Garlic Shrimp with Mixed Zucchini Noodles and Spaghetti
290 calories
Serves 2

The combination of zucchini noodles and spaghetti works really well here—giving the dish more body, while keeping the calories low.

2 oz whole wheat spaghetti
2 tbsp olive oil
1 small garlic clove, crushed
7 oz large raw frozen shrimp, thawed
2 medium zucchini, spiralized or very finely sliced (about 12 oz)
½ small lemon
Generous handful of fresh parsley or cilantro, chopped

1. Cook the spaghetti according to the package instructions, ensuring it remains al dente. Drain it, reserving the water.
2. Meanwhile, place the oil in a medium frying pan over medium heat. Add the garlic and sweat it for 30 seconds, then stir in the shrimp and cook for about 3 minutes, before adding the zucchini noodles.
3. Keep stirring for 2–3 minutes, and once the zucchini noodles start to soften, add the spaghetti to the pan with a generous squeeze of lemon juice and 1–2 tbsp of the reserved pasta water (or hot water) to loosen the mixture. Bring the pan to a gentle simmer, then immediately remove it from the heat.

4. Season it with some salt and plenty of freshly ground black pepper. Stir in the parsley and divide the mixture between 2 bowls.

LOWER CAL: For a lower-calorie version, skip the spaghetti and use larger zucchini (this reduces the calories by about 100 per person).

NONFAST DAY: Double the portion and add a large handful of salad leaves with a dressing such as Mint Mustard and Lime Dressing (page 201).

Sardines Roasted in Red and Yellow Peppers
220 calories
Serves 2

Canned sardines, while fantastically healthy, are not to everyone's taste. This is a delicious way of serving them, with the peppers providing a sweet and succulent foil to the salty fish.

2 red or yellow bell peppers, halved and seeded
3½ oz can sardines in olive oil
6 cherry tomatoes, halved
1 tbsp capers
2 garlic cloves, sliced
1 tbsp extra-virgin olive oil
2 slices of whole wheat sourdough, toasted (optional, add 144 calories)

1. Preheat the oven to 350°F.
2. Place the pepper halves on a small baking pan and divide the sardines between them. Drizzle the oil from the sardine can over the peppers.
3. Sprinkle over the tomatoes, capers, and garlic and some seasoning.
4. Place the pan in the oven for 15–20 minutes or until the peppers start to brown around the edges.
5. Serve two pepper halves on top of each slice of sourdough toast, if using.

TIP: Cans of sardines don't always contain the same amount of olive oil. You need a total of about 2 tbsp to drizzle into the peppers.

Mint Avocado and Chickpea Salad
350 calories
Serves 4

Chickpeas are a great source of complex carbohydrate (as well as protein), releasing slow-burn energy without spiking sugars.

For the salad:
2 avocados, pitted, peeled, and sliced
14 oz can chickpeas, drained (3 tbsp reserved liquid)
½ red onion, finely sliced
4 bok choy, trimmed and chopped
16 cherry tomatoes, halved
8 Brazil nuts, chopped

For the Mint Mustard and Lime Dressing:
Grated zest of 1 lime and juice of 2 limes
4 tbsp extra-virgin olive oil
1 tsp Dijon mustard
2 tbsp finely chopped mint

1. To make the dressing, whisk together the reserved chickpea liquid, lime zest and juice, oil, mustard, and mint. Season well.
2. Place all the salad ingredients except the nuts in a large bowl, pour over the dressing, and toss everything together.
3. Sprinkle the nuts on top and serve.

NONFAST DAY: Double the portion size.

Miso Eggplant "Steaks" with Roasted Carrots and Cashews

315 calories
Serves 2

Please don't be tempted to reduce the amount of olive oil in this recipe—this wonderful healthy fat gives this dish its rich taste and texture and will help keep you satiated for longer.

7 oz yellow and orange carrots, cut into batons
3 tbsp olive oil
1 oz cashews
1 eggplant, trimmed and sliced into "steaks,"
 ½ inch thick
2 tsp miso paste
Juice of ½ lime
4 oz fresh baby spinach

1. Preheat the oven to 400°F. Place the carrots in a baking pan and drizzle 1 tbsp of the oil over them. Roast them for 15–20 minutes or until they start to turn golden brown. Add the cashews for the last 5 minutes.
2. Meanwhile, spread both sides of the eggplant with miso paste. Place the remaining oil in a large nonstick frying pan over medium heat and gently fry the eggplant on both sides until they are lightly browned.
3. In the last few minutes of cooking, drizzle the lime juice over the eggplant. Then stir in the spinach, allowing it 1–2 minutes to wilt in the pan.

4. Finally, add the roasted carrots and some salt and freshly ground black pepper.

TIP: These eggplant "steaks," with their fabulous "umami" flavor, can be eaten with salads or any combination of cooked vegetables (32 calories on their own).

MORE SUBSTANTIAL: Add a green or colored leaf side salad (insignificant calories unless you add a dressing).

NONFAST DAYS: Add an extra eggplant "steak." Serve with boiled peas and a dollop of butter or a drizzle of olive oil. You might add 3 heaping tbsp cooked whole grains such as brown rice, or some legumes, such as puy lentils, from a package.

Mackerel, Beet, and Red Onion Salad
349 calories
Serves 4

Enjoy an omega-3 boost from this star of the oily fish group. We've made it even easier for you by using fish that has already been cooked and filleted.

1¼ lbs beets, trimmed, peeled, and cut into wedges
2 tbsp olive oil
1 tsp cumin seeds
2 red onions, cut into wedges
2 garlic cloves, finely chopped
3 smoked mackerel fillets, skinned and broken into large flakes (about 9 oz)
1 tbsp capers, coarsely chopped (optional)
1 tbsp apple cider vinegar
3–4 sprigs fresh dill or mint, chopped
Handful of fresh parsley, chopped
5 oz arugula or mixture of arugula and watercress

1. Preheat the oven to 400°F.
2. Place the beets in a roasting pan, drizzle with 1 tbsp oil, scatter the cumin seeds on top. Cover it with foil and roast for 45 minutes. Then discard the foil and stir in the onions and garlic. Cook the vegetables for another 15–20 minutes, or until they are tender.
3. Remove them from the oven and spoon them into a large bowl with the remaining ingredients. Toss everything together gently before serving.

MORE SUBSTANTIAL: Add 2 tbsp coarsely chopped toasted walnuts (80 calories).

NONFAST DAY: Add 2–3 heaping tbsp cooked brown rice or bulgur wheat.

Lentil, Pomegranate, and Feta Salad

395 calories
Serves 2

This colorful, flavorsome salad will keep you going through the day.

For the dressing:
2 tbsp extra-virgin olive oil
Juice of ½ lemon
1 tsp whole grain mustard

For the salad:
9 oz package cooked puy lentils
2 tbsp pomegranate seeds
½ cucumber, halved, seeded, and diced
4 oz feta cheese, diced
1 garlic clove, finely diced
6–8 fresh mint leaves, torn

1. Whisk the dressing ingredients together with some salt and freshly ground black pepper.
2. Place the lentils in a large bowl with the pomegranate seeds and cucumber, and crumble in the feta.
3. Stir in the diced garlic and torn mint leaves.
4. Pour the dressing over the lentil salad and toss everything together before serving.

MORE SUBSTANTIAL: Scatter 1 tbsp toasted flaked almonds or toasted hazelnuts on top (add about 100 calories). You might like to add a portion of sliced cold meats or smoked fish (see Extras on pages 243–45).

Pasta and Pesto Salad Jar
495 calories
Serves 1

This is the perfect way to enjoy a fresh, healthy, homemade salad when at work. All you need is a jar or container with a tight-fitting lid.

1½ tbsp pesto
2 tbsp cooled, cooked whole wheat pasta (pea or lentil pasta can be used as a gluten-free alternative)
2 oz fennel, finely sliced
3 oz cherry tomatoes, halved
1½ oz feta cheese, cut into cubes
Small handful of arugula or fresh baby spinach
1 tbsp pumpkin seeds, toasted

1. Spoon the pesto and cooked pasta into a container or a large glass jar and mix well.
2. Add the fennel and cherry tomatoes.
3. Stir in the feta, followed by the arugula and pumpkin seeds. Put the lid on and keep it in the fridge until it is needed (up to 24 hours).

TIP: Preferably use a jar with a wide mouth so it is easy to fill and to eat from, if you aren't transferring the salad to a plate.

MORE SUBSTANTIAL: For other tasty ingredients to add, see Extras on pages 243–45.

Pearl Barley and Pumpkin Seed Salad
340 calories
Serves 2

Pearl barley is a lovely whole grain with a smooth surface and slightly nutty flavor. It is great for mopping up sauces or dressing. And your microbiome will love it too.

For the dressing:
1 tbsp full-fat Greek yogurt
1 tbsp olive oil
Juice of 1 small lemon and zest of ½
1 small garlic clove, crushed
½ tbsp chopped fresh dill or mint

For the salad:
¼ cup pearl barley or pearled spelt
½ small red onion, finely chopped, or a handful
   of chives
1 tbsp toasted pumpkin seeds
1 tsp nigella or black sesame seeds
½ small apple, cored and diced

1. Mix the dressing ingredients together in a serving bowl with some salt and freshly ground black pepper.
2. Boil the barley in plenty of water according to the package instructions (usually about 40 minutes).
3. When the barley is cooked al dente, drain it and refresh it briefly under cold water. Stir it into

the dressing in the bowl, along with the onion, pumpkin seeds, nigella seeds, and apple.

NONFAST DAY: Add extra protein (see page 243) and make a double portion of salad.

Speedy Chinese Salmon Stir-Fry
360 calories
Serves 2

This really is a case of heat up the wok, throw in the ingredients, stir-fry, and serve.

1 tbsp coconut or rapeseed oil
½-inch piece fresh ginger, peeled and finely chopped or grated
8 oz package Chinese stir-fry vegetables
2 sweet chili cooked salmon fillets, flaked (about 6 oz), see Tip
1 tbsp dark soy sauce
½ tbsp mirin, Chinese wine, or sherry

1. Place a wok over high heat until it starts to smoke. Add the oil, immediately followed by the ginger, the vegetables, and a generous grinding of black pepper.
2. Stir-fry vigorously for a couple of minutes, then add the salmon.
3. Turn the heat down and add 1 tbsp water, the soy sauce, and the mirin. Keep stirring for a couple more minutes, until the vegetables are cooked but still crisp and the salmon is warmed through.
4. Remove the wok from the heat and serve.

TIP: If no sweet chili salmon is available, use cooked salmon fillets and sprinkle them with a pinch of red pepper flakes before adding them to the pan. For added flavor scatter a handful of chopped cilantro leaves and an extra ½ tsp red pepper flakes on top.

NONFAST DAY: Double the salmon portion, add a medium portion of whole wheat or soba noodles, and scatter 1 tbsp toasted sesame seeds and a handful of cashew nuts over the salmon and noodles.

MAIN MEALS

On the whole, these recipes are more substantial and some may take a bit longer to prepare than the light meals. It's up to you whether you have the main meal at lunchtime or in the evening. But in general, the earlier you eat your main meal, the better for your weight and metabolism.

Spanish Eggplant Stew with Chorizo
390 calories
Serves 2

A rich and nourishing stew, full of Mediterranean flavors.

3 tbsp olive oil
1 onion, diced
½ cup sliced cremini mushrooms
1 eggplant, diced
1 tsp mixed herbs
4 oz chorizo, diced
2 garlic cloves, sliced
14 oz can diced tomatoes

1. Sweat the onion in the oil in a casserole dish or saucepan with a lid over medium heat for 4–5 minutes, then add the mushrooms, eggplant, herbs, and chorizo.
2. Cook the mixture for 5 minutes, or until it starts to brown slightly, stirring frequently and adding the garlic for the last minute.
3. Pour in the tomatoes and ½ cup water (enough to loosen the mixture) and simmer for about 40 minutes, stirring occasionally.
4. Serve the stew with some steamed greens.

NONFAST DAY: Double the quantities, and serve with 2–3 heaping tbsp cooked brown rice or quinoa or throw in 2 handfuls of diced butternut squash along with the canned tomatoes.

Balsamic Fried Pork Chop with Garlicky White Bean Mash

470 calories
Serves 2

A juicy pork chop and mash with a twist.

For the mash (230 calories):
2 tbsp olive oil
1 small onion, diced
2 garlic cloves, diced
14 oz can cannellini beans or other white bean,
   liquid reserved
1-inch sprig fresh rosemary, leaves only, finely
   chopped

For the pork chop (240 calories):
½ tbsp olive oil
2 (7-oz) pork chops
1 tbsp balsamic vinegar

1. To make the mash, heat the oil in a saucepan
   and sauté the onion until it is translucent, about
   5 minutes. Add the garlic and cook for another
   minute, then stir in the beans with their liquid
   and cook them gently for 10 minutes, stirring
   occasionally.
2. Add the rosemary, a generous pinch of sea salt,
   and some freshly ground black pepper to the bean
   mixture and mash it vigorously.
3. Meanwhile, place a nonstick frying pan over
   medium heat, add the oil, and gently fry the pork

for 10–12 minutes, turning it once, until it is brown on both sides and the juices run clear.

4. Drizzle the balsamic vinegar over the steaks and serve them with the mash and a generous portion of Super-Simple Greens (page 235).

NONFAST DAY: Add another vegetable side dish such as Roasted Endive with Mustard and Walnuts (page 238).

Steak with Porcini Mushrooms
240 calories
Serves 2

Steak is an excellent source of protein and iron, while porcini mushrooms are high in fiber and very low in calories. Here they add a slightly sweet "foresty" taste to the sauce. A delicious combination.

½ oz dried porcini mushrooms
1 tbsp olive oil
1 large red onion, sliced
⅔ cup sliced cremini mushrooms
2 tsp cornstarch
2 (4-oz) sirloin steaks (see Tip)

1. Place the porcini mushrooms in a small bowl with just enough boiling water to cover them, and leave them to soak for 10 minutes.
2. Heat the oil in a frying pan and sauté the onion for 3 minutes, then add the sliced mushrooms. Cook over medium heat for another 4–5 minutes.
3. Stir in the cornstarch, followed by the porcini mushrooms and their soaking water. Continue to cook, stirring frequently, until the sauce thickens. If it looks too thick, add a little more water.
4. Meanwhile, cook the steaks to your liking, either on a grill or in a frying pan.
5. Serve the steaks with the mushroom sauce poured over them and some steamed green vegetables on the side.

TIP: We usually share 8 oz of steak (and don't worry about the few extra calories).

MORE SUBSTANTIAL: Add Creamy Cauli and White Bean Mash (page 239).

NONFAST DAY: Add some boiled or roasted carrots, and some olive oil on the steamed vegetables.

Low-Carb Stir-Fried Peppered Chicken
460 calories
Serves 2

A perfect light meal when you are in a hurry.

7 oz boneless, skinless chicken thighs, diced
2 tbsp soy sauce
½-inch piece fresh ginger, peeled and grated
2 tsp cornstarch
½ tsp Chinese five-spice powder
2 tbsp melted coconut or virgin rapeseed oil
8 oz package Chinese stir-fry vegetables
2 oz cashew nuts, toasted

1. Place the chicken in a nonmetallic bowl and add ½ tbsp of the soy sauce, along with the ginger, cornstarch, five-spice powder, and a generous grinding of black pepper. Mix everything together and leave it to marinate for 10 minutes.
2. In a pitcher, mix the remaining 1½ tbsp soy sauce with ½ cup hot water.
3. Heat the oil in a hot smoking wok or a large frying pan, then add the chicken. Stir-fry for 3–4 minutes, until it starts to brown and become opaque.
4. Reduce the heat to medium and mix in the vegetables, followed by the water and soy sauce mixture, and cook for another 2 minutes. Serve with the cashews scattered on top.

MORE SUBSTANTIAL: Serve it with Coconut Cauli Rice (page 228, add 105 calories) or konjac "Zero" noodles (page 190–91).

Sausage and Mushrooms with Spring Greens
545 calories
Serves 2

We love this one-pan dish, cooked with good-quality, meat-filled sausages. Yes, it contains quite a lot of calories, but there are still enough in hand for a breakfast or a light meal.

2 tbsp olive oil
4 good-quality pork sausages
1 onion, sliced
7 oz mushrooms, sliced
1 garlic clove, diced
7 oz spring greens, finely sliced
1 tbsp apple cider vinegar

1. Heat the oil in a large frying pan over medium heat, add the sausages and fry, turning them frequently until they start to brown.
2. Add the onion and mushrooms and continue to cook for 2–3 minutes, still stirring frequently.
3. Next, add the garlic, spring greens, and vinegar, along with 1–2 tbsp water.
4. Cover the pan and simmer for another 4–5 minutes, stirring occasionally.
5. Add some seasoning and serve with mustard on the side.

NONFAST DAY: Add 2–3 tbsp cooked puy lentils, quinoa, or pearl barley.

Chicken, Coconut, and Lentil Curry
360 calories
Serves 4

An easy go-to chicken curry, with lovely lentils to keep you and your microbiome in good nick.

2 tbsp coconut or virgin rapeseed oil
1 large onion, diced
1 tbsp curry powder
¾-inch piece fresh ginger, peeled and finely diced
4 boneless, skinless chicken thighs (1¼ lb), chopped into bite-size pieces
½ cup dried green lentils
1½ cups canned coconut milk
Juice of 2 limes
1 red or green bell pepper, seeded and sliced

1. Heat the oil in a medium saucepan and sauté the onion for 4–5 minutes.
2. Stir in the curry powder and ginger and cook for 1–2 minutes more, then add the chicken. Stir-fry for 2–3 minutes before pouring in the lentils, along with the coconut milk and lime juice.
3. Bring the mixture to a gentle boil, then reduce the heat, cover the pan, and simmer for 10 minutes, stirring occasionally, and adding some water if necessary.
4. Stir in the bell pepper and let the curry cook, with the lid on, for another 20 minutes.

MORE SUBSTANTIAL: Serve it with steamed snow peas or green beans (no significant calories) and Coconut Cauli Rice (page 228, add 105 calories).

NONFAST DAY: Serve it with 2–3 heaping tbsp cooked brown rice, some Raita (page 244) and a chopped hard-boiled egg.

Chili Lime Tuna with Beans and Diced Mango
490 calories
Serves 2

Cannellini beans are a healthy complex carbohydrate, not only good for reducing your blood sugars but also for nourishing your gut microbiome. Olive oil, which also has many health benefits, enhances the taste of all legumes and is fine on the calorie front when enjoyed as part of a relatively low-carb diet.

3 tbsp olive oil
1 garlic clove, diced
½ red chili, seeded and diced, or ½ tsp red pepper flakes
14 oz can cannellini beans, drained (2 tbsp liquid reserved)
Large bunch of fresh parsley, chopped
½ small red onion, very finely sliced
5 oz can tuna in oil, drained
Juice of 1 lime
½ small mango, peeled and finely diced
2 handfuls fresh baby spinach

1. Heat the oil in a frying pan and gently fry the garlic and chili for 1 minute. Add the beans and let them simmer for 2–3 minutes, stirring frequently.
2. Next, add the parsley, onion, tuna, and lime juice, along with 1–2 tbsp of the reserved bean liquid to loosen the mixture. Continue to cook it gently for a few more minutes until everything is heated through.

3. Stir in the mango.
4. Place a handful of spinach on each plate and serve the hot tuna and beans on top to wilt the spinach. Or wilt the spinach for 1–2 minutes in the microwave before adding the tuna mixture.

TIPS: Although mango is a fairly high-sugar fruit, it has lots of fiber, and eating it with a meal reduces any sugar spike. In some people with IBS, legumes such as beans can make symptoms worse—in which case it may be best to introduce them gradually.

MORE SUBSTANTIAL: Serve it with a crisp green salad, or steamed green vegetables (no extra calories unless you add a dressing).

Peppered Roasted Cod with Nutty Broccoli
430 calories
Serves 2

Full of nutrients, crunch, and fiber—and utterly delicious.

9 oz broccoli, cut into long florets (including
    the stalk)
1 oz hazelnuts, chopped
2 (5-oz) cod loins or any white fish fillets
½ tbsp ground almonds
1½ tbsp olive oil
Squeeze of lemon juice to serve

1. Preheat the oven to 350°F.
2. Place the broccoli in a roasting pan, cover it with foil, and roast it for 5 minutes.
3. Remove the pan from the oven, discard the foil, and nestle the fish among the broccoli florets. Scatter the nuts over the broccoli. Then sprinkle 1 tsp of freshly ground black pepper and some sea salt over the fish. Drizzle with the oil.
4. Return the pan to the oven for 10–12 minutes, or until the fish is cooked through, the broccoli is slightly charred, and the nuts are golden.
5. Serve with a generous squeeze of lemon juice.

MORE SUBSTANTIAL: Add 3–4 oz spinach, wilted, or a green and colored leaf salad (only add extra calories if you use a dressing—see page 244).

NONFAST DAY: Add some spinach steamed with 1 tsp butter or ½ tbsp extra-virgin olive oil, and 2–3 heaping tbsp cooked quinoa or brown rice.

Haddock Steamed with Thai Spices
300 calories
Serves 1

Bok choy is an excellent probiotic that promotes a
healthy microbiome.

2 bok choy, chopped
½ red bell pepper, seeded and chopped
2 green onions, trimmed
1 lemongrass stalk, halved and bruised (optional)
¼-inch piece fresh ginger, peeled and sliced
1 garlic clove, sliced
5 oz haddock fillet or other white fish
2–3 sprigs fresh cilantro
2 tsp rice wine, mirin, or sherry
1 tsp soy sauce
1 tbsp olive oil

1. Place the bok choy, bell pepper, and green onions
   in a steamer.
2. Lay the lemongrass (if using), ginger, and garlic on
   a large square of parchment paper and place the
   haddock on top. Scatter the cilantro, rice wine, and
   some salt and pepper over the surface.
3. Loosely fold the parchment to encase the fish and
   herbs and lay it on top of the vegetables in the
   steamer.
4. Steam it for 5–6 minutes, or until the fish is cooked
   through.
5. Serve the fish on top of the vegetables, drizzled
   with the juices from the parchment paper, the oil,
   and soy sauce.

TIP: If you don't have a pan with a steamer tray, place the wrapped fish and vegetables in a baking dish. Pour 2–3 tbsp water in the base of the dish, cover it with a lid or foil, then steam it in a preheated oven at 350°F for 8–10 minutes or until the vegetables are tender and the fish cooked through.

NONFAST DAY: Double the portion and serve with some whole wheat or soba noodles.

Shrimp Korma with Coconut Cauli Rice
320 calories
Serves 4

A popular, creamy curry with a delicate flavor and rich in healthy fats.

For the rice:
1 large head cauliflower, cut into florets
1 tbsp coconut oil
1 tbsp desiccated coconut

For the korma:
1 tbsp coconut oil
2 large onions, diced
4 garlic cloves, sliced
¾-inch piece fresh ginger, peeled and diced
3 tbsp korma paste
1¾ cups coconut milk
14 oz frozen large shrimp, peeled, deveined, and thawed
Large handful of fresh spinach leaves
2 tbsp full-fat Greek yogurt
2 tbsp fresh cilantro, chopped

1. Blitz the cauliflower in a food processor until it has a ricelike consistency.
2. Heat the oil in a wok or frying pan and add the cauliflower and desiccated coconut.
3. Fry the mixture over low heat, stirring occasionally, for 10–12 minutes, or until the cauliflower is tender but still al dente.
4. Heat the oil in a saucepan over low heat and sauté

the onions, garlic, and ginger for 8–10 minutes, or until they are lightly golden.

5. Add the korma paste and after a minute, pour in the coconut milk. Bring it to a boil, then reduce the heat, and simmer for 8–10 minutes, by which time the sauce should have reduced and thickened.

6. Remove the pan from the heat and, using a handheld blender, blitz the sauce until it is smooth.

7. Return it to the heat and add the shrimp. Let them simmer gently in the sauce for 3–4 minutes, then stir in the spinach, yogurt, and some seasoning.

8. Scatter the cilantro on top of the curry and serve with the Coconut Cauli Rice.

TIP: You can swap the shrimp for cooked diced chicken (see Extras on pages 243–45 for swaps)

MORE SUBSTANTIAL: Serve it with snow peas or thin green beans and 2 tbsp Raita (page 244).

Vegan Rogan Josh
310 calories
Serves 4

Yes, you can still enjoy eating curry ... just skip the potato, white rice, naan, and chapattis!

3 tbsp olive oil
2 onions, 1 sliced in rings, the other chopped
10 oz butternut squash, peeled and chopped
3 garlic cloves, sliced
½ red bell pepper, seeded and sliced
7 oz portobello mushrooms, chopped
14 oz can chickpeas, drained
2 tbsp rogan josh paste
14 oz can diced tomatoes
Handful of kale
2 tbsp chopped fresh cilantro

1. Heat the oil in a saucepan over medium heat and sauté the onion rings for about 8–10 minutes, or until they are golden and slightly crispy. Remove them from the pan and set aside.
2. Using the same pan and oil, sauté the chopped onions for 2–3 minutes. Add the butternut squash, garlic, bell peppers, and mushrooms and cook for another 3–4 minutes.
3. Stir in the chickpeas with the rogan josh paste, followed by the tomatoes.
4. Cover the pan and simmer for 15 minutes, or until the vegetables are tender. Add water if necessary to loosen the sauce.

5. Stir in the kale and cook for 2 minutes, then add the cilantro and some seasoning. Garnish the curry with the onion rings and serve with Coconut Cauli Rice (page 228, add 105 calories).

MORE SUBSTANTIAL: Add 1 tbsp toasted cashew nuts (20g, add 115 calories).

NONFAST DAY: Double the portion. You could have 2–3 heaping tbsp cooked brown rice instead of the Coconut Cauli Rice.

Turmeric Roasted Cauliflower with Dal
414 calories
Serves 4

Satisfyingly filling and delivering a rich burst of flavor. Don't be put off by the long list of ingredients—they are all likely to be in your store cupboard. It's such an easy dish to prepare too.

For the cauliflower:
1 large head cauliflower, sliced into ¾-inch-thick "steaks"
1 tbsp olive oil
1 tsp ground turmeric
1 garlic clove, thinly sliced

For the dal:
½ tbsp coconut oil
1 onion, diced
½–1 red chili, seeded and finely diced
1 tsp cumin seeds
2 garlic cloves, crushed
1 tbsp medium curry powder
8 oz red lentils
14 oz can light coconut milk
1¾ cups vegetable stock
Generous handful of spinach leaves
2 tbsp chopped fresh cilantro (optional)
Juice of ½ lemon
2 tbsp flaked almonds, toasted

1. Preheat the oven to 400°F. Place the cauliflower and any remaining florets in a large roasting pan and sprinkle the olive oil over them.
2. Roast them for 15 minutes, then remove them from the oven and scatter over the turmeric and garlic. Return them to the oven for another 10–15 minutes, or until they start to brown.
3. Meanwhile, heat the coconut oil in a lidded saucepan and gently fry the onion and chili for 3–4 minutes.
4. Add the cumin, garlic, and curry powder and cook for another 1–2 minutes before stirring in the lentils, followed by the coconut milk and stock. Cover the pan and simmer for 15 minutes, or until the lentils are soft.
5. Add the spinach and once it has wilted, stir in the cilantro, if using, and some seasoning.
6. Squeeze the lemon over the cauliflower. Serve it topped with the dal and the flaked almonds.

TIP: Make double the quantity of dal and freeze the extra portions.

NONFAST DAY: Serve it with some Raita (page 244) and a portion of Vegan Rogan Josh (page 230).

VEGETABLE SIDES AND SWAPS

We believe that most people would benefit significantly from increasing their intake of nonstarchy vegetables, with all the health-promoting phytonutrients and gut-friendly roughage they contain. Feel free to add steamed leafy greens whenever you want—even with a teaspoonful of butter or coconut or olive oil (see page opposite), which enhance the taste considerably, while increasing the calorie count by only a small amount.

With starchy vegetables, you need to be more cautious, in particular with potatoes and sweet potatoes. These are carb storage devices, and should be eaten only in small quantities, if at all, while you are on this diet. See page 239 for a delicious mashed potato substitute.

Super-Simple Greens 2 Ways
Serves 1, and NO calorie counting

Simple Steamed Cabbage:
4 oz finely sliced cabbage
½ tsp butter or olive oil
¼ tsp nigella seeds or black sesame seeds (optional)

Steam the cabbage briefly for 3–4 minutes or until it starts to soften. Place it in a dish, stir in the butter, and season it well with salt and freshly ground black pepper. Add the seeds, if using.

Sizzling Stir-Fried Spring Greens:
1 tsp rapeseed or coconut oil
1 tsp grated or diced fresh ginger
3 cups spring greens, finely sliced
Dash of soy sauce

1. Place the oil in a wok or large frying pan over medium to high heat and stir in the ginger. Add the greens and sauté them until they start to soften, 2–3 minutes.
2. Season them well with salt and plenty of freshly ground black pepper.

Instant Vegetable Stir-Fry
210 calories
Serves 1

This is an excellent, no-fuss way to get your vegetables, either as a light meal on its own or as a side dish.

1 tbsp rapeseed or coconut oil
5 oz Chinese stir-fry vegetables
1 small garlic clove, crushed
⅛-inch piece fresh ginger, diced or grated
½ tbsp soy sauce

1. Heat the wok on high until it starts to smoke, drizzle in the oil, and add the vegetables.
2. Reduce the heat to medium and stir in the garlic and ginger. Stir-fry the vegetables for no more than 2–3 minutes to ensure they retain their crunch.
3. Stir 1 tbsp water and the soy sauce into the vegetables and toss for 30 seconds. Serve immediately.

TIP: Don't worry about variations in the calorie counts of different vegetable stir-fry packages. They are healthy calories, many of which won't even be broken down for energy but will feed the microbiome farther down in the gut.

MORE SUBSTANTIAL: Add 1 or more of the following along with the vegetables: 1 oz cashew nuts (172 calories), 2 tsp sesame seeds (60 calories), 3.5 oz tofu (73 calories), 3.5 oz cooked chicken (153 calories), 3.5 oz frozen shrimp, thawed (79 calories). For more Extras, see pages 243–45.

Quick Pickled Fennel and Radishes

Superfast and easy to make, and very low in calories. Pile it on top of fish or use it to pep up a salad.

½ fennel bulb, trimmed
4 radishes, trimmed
2 tsp raw organic apple cider vinegar
1 tsp mirin, Chinese wine, or sherry (optional)

1. Place the fennel and radishes cut side down and slice them very finely, if possible with a mandoline. If you don't have a mandoline, cut the radishes in half lengthwise first to make them easier to slice into half-moon shapes.
2. Place the fennel and radishes in a bowl with the vinegar and mirin, if using. Add a generous pinch of sea salt and massage it into the vegetables for a few minutes. Leave them to marinate for up to 30 minutes for the best flavor.
3. Drain the liquid before eating.

TIP: This pickle can be kept in the fridge for up to 24 hours. Please note that it does not boost the gut-friendly bacteria in the same way as the sauerkraut dishes on pages 240–41. To obtain this benefit, the vegetables need to ferment for longer.

Roasted Endive with Mustard and Walnuts
290 calories
Serves 2 (or 4 as a side)

With the smoky bitterness of charred endive, the tang of mustard, and the crunch of walnuts, this dish is a mouthwatering combination of textures and flavors. And your microbiome will love it, as endive is full of the prebiotic inulin.

4 medium endive (red if available), halved lengthwise
2 tbsp olive oil
2 tsp whole grain mustard
1 tbsp coarsely chopped walnuts
1 tbsp grated Parmesan

1. Preheat the oven to 375°F. Place the endive cut side up in a medium ovenproof baking dish.
2. Combine the oil and mustard in a small bowl, then spread it over the endive.
3. Cover the baking dish with foil and place it in the oven for 15–20 minutes.
4. Remove it from the oven and sprinkle with the walnuts, Parmesan, and a generous grinding of black pepper.
5. Bake for another 10 minutes, or until the endive starts to brown around the edges.

MORE SUBSTANTIAL: Add a large handful of baby spinach to each plate and place the endive on top to wilt the spinach, or wilt it for a few minutes in a nonstick pan first.

NONFAST DAY: Add 2–3 heaping tbsp cooked brown rice or quinoa. Or serve the endive as a side with another dish, such as Steak with Porcini Mushrooms (page 216), or Peppered Roasted Cod with Nutty Broccoli (page 224).

Creamy Cauli and White Bean Mash
160 calories
Serves 4

This delicious mash makes a great substitute for starchy potatoes. Not only will it keep you full for longer but it will produce less of a sugar spike—both important factors in weight loss.

1 small head cauliflower, cut into small florets
7 oz canned cannellini beans, drained, 2 tbsp liquid reserved
2 oz cheddar cheese, chopped
2 tbsp olive oil

1. Steam the cauliflower and beans for 10–12 minutes, or until the cauliflower is tender.
2. Transfer them to a food processor with the remaining ingredients and blend them until you have a smooth mixture, adding 1–2 tbsp of the liquid from the beans to loosen the mash if necessary. Season it well with salt and freshly ground black pepper.

White Cabbage and Red Onion Sauerkraut 2 Ways

Home fermenting is quick, easy, fun, and cheap, and your gut microbiome will love it! Here are 2 versions of fermented cabbage, which both offer delicious sweet, salty, and tangy flavors with a slight crunch. They go well with almost any savory food.

Sauerkraut with Caraway Seeds
180 calories (whole recipe)

This is a classic sauerkraut that provides plenty of flavor but adds minimal calories. We love the hint of caraway, but feel free to experiment with other seeds such as cumin, toasted coriander, or mustard. Add it to dishes for extra flavor, as you would a pickle.

½ medium head white cabbage, quartered lengthwise, hard core removed, finely sliced
1½ red onions, halved and sliced
1 tsp caraway seeds
½ tbsp sea salt or kosher salt
2 (8-oz) clean jam jars with tight-fitting lids

1. Mix the cabbage, onions, and caraway seeds together in a large bowl, sprinkling the salt between the layers as you fill it. Massage the salt into the vegetables. Leave it for 1–2 hours.
2. Spoon the cabbage mixture and the juices into the jars.

3. Pack the mixture in the jars, pressing it down. Leave ⅛–¼-inch headspace. If there is not enough liquid to cover the mixture you can top up either with a few teaspoonfuls of filtered water or brine (made with 1 tsp sea salt dissolved in ¾ cup filtered water).

4. You can use a stone or piece of ceramic to keep the vegetables submerged. Place the sealed jars on a plate to catch any overflow. Keep them at room temperature, out of direct sunlight. For the first few days, open the jars daily and press down the contents, to release the bubbles formed by the sauerkraut. Then repeat this process every few days for 1–2 weeks (usually about 1 week will do) until it is fermented to your taste.

5. Store the jars in the fridge for 2–3 months.

Mild Kimchi-Style Sauerkraut
220 calories (whole recipe)

Otherwise known as Asian sauerkraut, this spicy, exotic, strongly flavored fermented vegetable dish is the core of Korean cuisine. This recipe is a milder version.

½ medium head white cabbage, quartered lengthwise, hard core removed, sliced into ⅛–¾-inch ribbons
1½ red onions, halved and sliced
½ tbsp sea salt or kosher salt
2 tsp grated garlic
1 tsp grated fresh ginger
1 tsp sugar

1 tbsp fish or soy sauce
2–4 tsp red pepper flakes, or to taste
1 tsp sweet paprika
2 (8-oz) clean jam jars with tight-fitting lids

1. Mix the cabbage with the onions in a large bowl,
   sprinkling the salt between the layers as you fill it.
   Massage the salt into the vegetables. Let stand for
   about 2 hours.
2. Stir in the garlic and ginger and mix well.
3. Follow steps 2–5 of Sauerkraut with Caraway
   Seeds (page 240) and add the extra step below.
4. After 3–4 days, gently mix in the rest of the
   ingredients (the cabbage doesn't ferment effectively
   with the spices, so these can be added a bit later in
   the process).

TIP: Eat it with an omelet or cold meat, scatter it on fish,
salads, stew, or soups.

And for those little extras . . .

Many of the recipes include suggestions for how to adapt a dish for a nonfast day or to make it more substantial. Here are some further suggestions for how to increase protein content or make a meal more satiating.

- 1 tbsp chopped fried bacon (23 calories)
- 1 tbsp chopped chorizo (29 calories)
- 1.4 oz sliced mushrooms, fried in 1 tsp olive oil for 4–5 minutes (63 calories)
- 1 tbsp grated cheese (41 calories)
- 1 oz halloumi, sliced and lightly fried in 1 tsp olive oil (145 calories)
- 1.5 oz tuna, canned in oil (85 calories)
- Handful of nuts (½ tbsp each of walnuts, almonds, hazelnuts, 195 calories)
- 2.5 oz cooked chicken breast (115 calories)
- 2.5 oz frozen shrimp, thawed (59 calories)
- 3.5 oz tofu (73 calories)
- 2 tsp sesame seeds (60 calories)
- 1 tbsp full-fat Greek yogurt—it's worth the extra calories! (37 calories)
- 1 oz cheddar cheese, matchbox-sized piece (124 calories)
- Crispy fried onion rings for 2 people: heat 1 tbsp olive oil and sauté 1 small onion sliced into rings, turning them frequently until they are golden and slightly crispy (60 calories per serving)

- Raita for 2 people: mix 4 tbsp full-fat Greek yogurt with ¼ small cucumber, grated, and a pinch of cumin seeds in a small bowl (97 calories per serving)
- Olive oil and apple cider vinegar dressing for 2 people: whisk 2 tbsp extra-virgin olive oil with 1 tbsp raw cider vinegar and some salt and freshly ground black pepper (100 calories per serving). Dressings are not just for salads; they are a great way to liven up broccoli and leafy greens.
- Drizzle of olive oil. Use good-quality extra-virgin olive oil if you can and don't worry about counting the calories in the odd teaspoonful here or there--oil makes food taste great and your body needs it for vitamins and energy. Remember, *fat does not make you fat*!

Whole grains and legumes

Although moderately high in calories, whole grains and legumes, such as brown rice and lentils, are complex carbs and contain beneficial quantities of fiber that feed the microbiome in your gut, leading to the production of substances that reduce inflammation, lower blood sugars, and improve health. We recommend cooking grains and legumes in larger batches to be frozen in portions. Crumble in half a stock cube during cooking for added flavor.

Legumes are also a particularly good source of protein for vegetarians. Add 2 heaping tbsp on a fast day, and up to 3 on a nonfast day.

- Cooked brown rice (21 calories per 1 tbsp)
- Cooked quinoa (18 calories per 1 tbsp)
- Cooked bulgar wheat (13 calories per 1 tbsp)
- Cooked puy lentils (18 calories per 1 tbsp)
- Cooked pearl barley (19 calories per 1 tbsp)

OCCASIONAL TREATS

Fast days are not all about deprivation, so we've included some (modest) treats, ideally to be enjoyed immediately after a meal when they will cause less of a blood sugar spike and be less likely to be stored as fat. Eating these treats between meals will raise your blood sugars, which will in turn increase insulin production and stop your body from burning fats.

Stewed Rhubarb and Ginger
40 calories
Serves 4

Juicy, pleasantly tart, with bursts of sweet ginger, and positively overflowing with vitamins C and K.

14 oz rhubarb, trimmed and diced into ¼–¾-inch pieces
Juice of ½ orange
3 knobs of stem ginger in syrup, drained and diced

1. Place all the ingredients in a small pan and bring to a boil. Cover and let simmer for 2–3 minutes to soften the rhubarb.
2. Serve hot, cold, or in between, with 1 tbsp full-fat Greek yogurt (add 37 calories) or a dairy-free equivalent such as coconut yogurt.

TIP: If, like Michael, you or anyone in your household is addicted to stem ginger, keep it, preferably out of sight, at the back of the fridge! Fill the freezer with uncooked diced rhubarb when it's in season as it keeps well.

MORE SUBSTANTIAL: Add a small handful of nuts (about ½ oz, 100 calories).

Banana and Cranberry Lunchbox Bars
195 calories per bar
Makes 12

Perfect to take to work for lunch or grab as an occasional breakfast substitute if you're running late.

1¾ oz soft dates
2 unripe bananas
⅓ cup coconut oil, melted
¼ cup rolled oats
1½ cups ground almonds
⅔ cup dried cranberries
⅔ cup pecans, chopped

1. Preheat the oven to 400°F. Grease and line an 8-inch square baking pan with parchment paper.
2. Simmer the dates in ½ cup water in a small pan for about 10 minutes, or until they have softened and most of the water has evaporated.
3. Blitz the dates with the bananas in a food processor or with a handheld blender until you have a smoothish paste. Transfer it to a bowl and stir in the oil. Add the oats, almonds, cranberries, and pecans and mix well.
4. Pour the mixture into the prepared pan, pressing it down into the corners and leveling the top with the back of a spoon.
5. Bake for 20–22 minutes, or until the top is lightly golden. Cut into bars while it is still warm and let cool for 10 minutes. Remove the bars from the pan

and store them in an airtight container for up to 5 days, or in the freezer.

TIP: Any dried fruit works well in this recipe. You can substitute the almonds with chopped hazelnuts or walnuts.

Mango Chia Rice Pudding
149 calories
Serves 4

Comfort food with a healthy twist—and a great way to use up leftover brown rice.

3 tbsp cooked brown rice
1 tsp vanilla extract
Seeds of 3 cardamom pods
1½ cups canned coconut milk
½ tbsp maple syrup (optional)
1 tbsp chia seeds
1 ripe mango, peeled and finely diced

1. Put all the ingredients except the mango in a small saucepan over a low heat.
2. Bring the mixture to a simmer and cook for 18–20 minutes, or until it is thick and creamy. Stir frequently and add a little water to loosen it, if necessary.
3. Stir in most of the mango, leaving a few pieces to scatter on top. Serve the pudding warm, or leave it in the fridge to enjoy cold.

TIP: Delicious with black or red rice but needs cooking for 5–10 minutes longer.

NONFAST DAY: Scatter a handful of chopped toasted walnuts, almonds, or hazelnuts on top before serving.

Chili Chocolate Thins with Pistachio Crunch

75 calories
Serves 6-8

These chocolate treats have a thrilling chili kick. They're ideal to nibble after a meal or to scatter over strawberries or raspberries.

3 oz dark chocolate, at least 70% cocoa solids, chopped
Pinch of chili powder
2 tbsp chopped toasted pistachio nuts

1. Spread an 8 × 12-inch piece of parchment paper (or a piece of non-PVC plastic wrap) on the base of a baking tray, or a silicone baking mat.
2. Melt the chocolate in a bowl over a pan of gently simmering water, stirring frequently. Or use a microwave: pulse on high, stirring the chocolate every 30 seconds or so for about 2 minutes.
3. Stir in the chili, then pour the chocolate over the parchment. Tip the tray so the chocolate spreads out to form a very thin sheet, or use a palette knife to even it out.
4. Scatter the pistachio nuts over the chocolate and cool, ideally in the fridge.
5. Once it is completely set, break it into pieces.

GOOD HYDRATION

These drinks contain insignificant calories and anyway, let's face it, you can't count everything . . .

Keeping well hydrated is vital for maintaining energy levels and helping to reduce hunger pangs. Odd as it might sound, people commonly confuse mild thirst with hunger. And by the time you are thirsty, you are already slightly dehydrated. So it's important to keep ahead of the game.

Most people need an extra ½–1 quart of water on 800 days, when they are not only missing out on the fluid they would usually get in their meals, but also losing water in the process of burning fat—even more so in hot weather or with vigorous exercise.

These drinks also give you something interesting to sip when you are eking out the time before the next meal.

Flavored or carbonated water

Add very thin slices of cucumber, mint, quartered strawberries, lemon, lime . . . or any combination of these to water. The longer you can leave the water to steep in the fridge, the more flavor it will acquire.

Herbal/fruit teas—can be drunk hot or cold
Serves 1

Green tea: Just place a tea bag in a mug and pour some hot water over it. Add extra flavor with a squeeze of lemon.

Ginger tea with turmeric: Place a tea bag in a mug with a very thin slice of ginger and ¼-inch finely sliced turmeric (no need to peel them). You can also try 2 drops of vanilla extract for some added flavor. Top it up with boiling water and allow it to brew for at least 5 minutes. This tea is best taken after a meal, as fatty food massively increases absorption of curcumin, the active ingredient in turmeric that contributes to the anti-inflammatory and immunity-boosting properties.

Minted lemon tea: Place a handful of fresh mint leaves (or a mint tea bag) in a mug with a generous squeeze of lemon juice. Pour over some boiling water and allow it to brew for at least 5 minutes.

Fresh herb infusion: Add a small handful of any fresh herbs such as thyme, basil, rosemary, sage, or oregano to a mug, or use dried herbal tea. Pour over some boiling water and allow it to brew for at least 5 minutes. Try out various combinations to find your perfect blend.

Herbal teas: Keep a few types of herbal teas in your cupboard, such as mint, peppermint, chamomile, rooibos, jasmine, or any of the wild and wonderful variations available to keep your taste buds firing.

FAST800 MENUS

All these suggested menus add up to around 800 calories a day. Don't obsess too much about the exact calories as the reality is that the amount we absorb varies from person to person and depends on the nature of the food we are eating. Pick and choose from the planners, whether you are doing the Very Fast800 or the New 5:2, and feel free to swap meals around and have your main meal for lunch and vice versa. Calories, if you need them, are on the recipe pages.

Meal planner for 3 meals a day—week 1

Day	Breakfast
1	Easy Bacon and Egg Muffins (page 172)
2	Speedy Eggs and Avocado (page 175)
3	Creamy Green Smoothie (page 177)
4	Porridge with Pistachio and Chia (page 174)
5	Boiled Eggs with Spiced Asparagus Soldiers (page 171)
6	Turmeric Spiced Mushroom Omelet (page 184)
7	Baked Salmon and Eggs with Chives (page 173)

Lunch	Dinner
Hummus in a Hurry (page 179)	Chicken Coconut and Lentil Curry (page 220)
Sliced Ham with Purple Slaw (page 186)	Shrimp Korma with Coconut Cauli Rice (page 228)
Dark Rye Bread with Egg and Spinach (page 183)	Steak with Porcini Mushrooms (page 216)
Sardines Roasted in Red and Yellow Peppers (page 200)	Vegan Rogan Josh (page 230)
Root Vegetables and Turmeric Soup (page 194)	Spanish Eggplant Stew with Chorizo (page 213)
Quick 'n' Easy Pea and Spinach Soup (page 193)	Low-Carb Stir-Fried Peppered Chicken (page 218)
Instant Miso Soup with Mushrooms and Greens (page 192)	Sausage with Mushrooms and Spring Greens (page 219)

Meal planner for 3 meals a day—week 2

Day	Breakfast
8	Spiced Mango Smoothie (page 177)
9	Porridge with Pistachios and Chia (page 174)
10	Boiled Egg with Spiced Asparagus Soldiers (page 171)
11	Turmeric Spiced Mushroom Omelet (page 184)
12	Baked Salmon and Eggs with Chives (page 173)
13	Tomato and Basil Omelet (page 176)
14	Speedy Eggs and Avocado (page 175)

Lunch	Dinner
Minced Pork and Snow Pea Stir-Fry with Noodles (page 190)	Haddock Steamed with Thai Spices (page 226)
Tapenade with Feta (page 180)	Speedy Chinese Salmon Stir-Fry (page 210)
Red Lentil and Coconut Soup (page 195)	Shrimp Korma with Coconut Cauli Rice (page 228)
Pasta and Pesto Salad Jar (page 207)	Tapenade with Feta (page 180)
Crunchy Zucchini Canapés 3 Ways (page 181)	Garlic Shrimp with Mixed Zucchini Noodles and Spaghetti (page 198)
Roasted Endive with Mustard and Walnuts (page 238)	Mackerel, Beet, and Red Onion Salad (page 204)
Miso Eggplant "Steaks" with Carrots and Cashews (page 202)	Lemon and Thyme Chicken Kebabs (page 188)

Meal planner for 2 meals a day—week 1

Day	Breakfast
1	Smashed Avocado on Dark Rye Bread (page 182)
2	–
3	Baked Salmon and Eggs with Chives (page 173)
4	–
5	Speedy Eggs and Avocado (page 175) and 1 Banana and Cranberry Lunchbox Bar (page 248)
6	–
7	Porridge with Pistachios and Chia (page 174)

Lunch	Dinner
–	Sausage and Mushrooms with Spring Greens (page 219)
Chili Lime Tuna with Beans and Diced Mango (page 222)	Shrimp Korma with Coconut Cauli Rice (page 228)
–	Low-Carb Stir-Fried Peppered Chicken (page 218)
Lentil, Pomegranate, and Feta Salad (page 206)	Balsamic Fried Pork Chop with Garlicky White Bean Mash (page 214)
–	Spanish Eggplant Stew with Chorizo (page 213)
Mackerel, Beet, and Red Onion Salad (page 204)	Peppered Roast Cod and Nutty Broccoli (page 224)
–	Turmeric Roasted Cauliflower with Dal (page 232)

Meal planner for 2 meals a day—week 2

Day	Breakfast
8	–
9	Porridge with Pistachios and Chia (page 174)
10	–
11	Baked Salmon and Eggs with Chives (page 173)
12	–
13	Porridge with Pistachios and Chia (page 174)
14	–

Lunch	Dinner
Pearl Barley and Pumpkin Seed Salad (page 208)	Peppered Roast Cod with Nutty Broccoli (page 224)
–	Speedy Chinese Salmon Stir-Fry (page 210)
Pasta and Pesto Salad Jar (page 207)	Shrimp Korma with Coconut Cauli Rice (page 228)
–	Low-Carb Stir-Fried Peppered Chicken (page 218)
Mint Avocado and Chickpea Salad (page 201)	Sausage and Mushrooms with Spring Greens (page 219)
–	Chicken Coconut and Lentil Curry (page 220)
Easy Bacon and Egg Muffins (page 172) with Red Lentil and Coconut Soup (page 195)	Minced Pork and Snow Pea Stir-Fry with Noodles (page 190)

Some Quick Notes on the "Scientific Method"

One of the things people find so confusing about health advice is that it seems to keep on changing. One moment fat is bad for us, the next it's good. Not so long ago we were told that because eggs are rich in cholesterol we should avoid them. Now we're told eggs are full of high-quality protein and are a great way to start the day.

Why does this happen? And how can you decide where the truth lies?

Nutritional science, like any form of science, changes in response to new studies. But there are levels of "proof," with some sorts of evidence being more reliable than others. Here's a quick rundown, from the weakest to the strongest sources of evidence (with 1 being weak and 4 being strong).

1. Animal studies (weak evidence)

Animals, like rats and mice, are often used to test new diets and new ideas. Using small animals in experiments is cheap and it is often a good starting point for trying to understand how a particular food or chemical might affect humans. But animal studies can also be misleading, and this is one of the reasons why there are so many conflicting claims in the media. Just because something is good or bad for a rat, doesn't automatically mean the same for a human.

I remember reading claims that drinking coffee causes cancer. That belief was based almost entirely on animal studies where rats were given huge and unrealistic doses of some of the chemicals you find in roasted coffee, like acrylamide. The World Health Organization says acrylamide "probably causes cancer."

So should you be putting down that cup of coffee? Absolutely not. Multiple human studies have shown that you get a wide range of benefits from drinking coffee. A recent review[41] found that regular coffee drinkers have a lower risk of developing liver, prostate, and colon cancer, as well as type 2 diabetes, Parkinson's, and heart disease. The more coffee you drink—up to three or four cups a day—the greater the benefits.

Roasted coffee can contain tiny amounts of acrylamide, but it also contains over 1,000 other natural chemicals, many of which have antioxidant, anti-inflammatory, or anticancer properties. The only people who really need to be careful about the amount of coffee they drink are pregnant women, as there is some evidence that drinking a lot of coffee is linked to the risk of a small baby, early birth, or even miscarriage.

In this book I have been quoting animal studies, but I have tried, where possible, to back them up with human studies.

2. Government guidelines (somewhat weak)

Government guidelines are the next weakest form of evidence, because they are often out of date and based on incomplete science.

The current epidemic of peanut allergy, a serious and

sometimes fatal condition, is partly the result of well-meaning government advice issued decades ago. When Clare was pregnant with our first son she was told to avoid peanuts and to avoid giving him peanuts when he was young. It seemed to make sense that if kids aren't exposed to peanuts they won't become sensitized.

That advice turned out to be completely wrong, which is why current advice is now exactly the opposite.

Studies done over the last 10 years have shown that whether a pregnant woman eats peanuts or not makes no difference to the child's risk developing an allergy.

In fact, we now know that giving very young children food to eat containing peanuts (from the age of four months onwards) will actually cut their risk of developing a peanut allergy later in life. Ironically, giving young children peanuts is particularly important if they have a genetic risk, i.e., if their parents have a peanut allergy.

Another example of well-meaning government advice that turned out to have terrible consequences is the low-fat message, heavily promoted by governments around the world since the early 1980s. Well, it seemed obvious, eating fat makes you fat, and like pouring fat down the drain it blocks it, so the fat must be blocking people's arteries too . . .

The low-fat message was always a bit more complex than "fat is bad and carbs are good," but that is how it was widely interpreted—healthy fats, like milk, yogurt, eggs, oily fish, and nuts, were demonized. Instead, food manufacturers seized the chance to cram their products with starchy foods and sugar, then sell them as "healthy" because they were "fat-free" or "cholesterol-free."

Despite being based on weak science and decades of evidence to the contrary, the low-fat message is still constantly regurgitated.

3. Cohort studies (moderately strong)

Much of what we now believe about "healthy eating" is based on cohort studies. This is where you take a group of people with something in common (like being health professionals), get them to do lots of tests and fill in questionnaires, and then follow them over time to see what happens to them.

A good example of this is The Health Professionals Follow-up Study[42] that started in 1986. It consists of 51,529 dentists, pharmacists, osteopaths, and vets who were middle-aged at the beginning of the study.

Among other things this study has shown is that those who eat a Mediterranean-style diet have fewer problems with memory as they get older.

4. Randomized controlled trials (strong evidence)

The weakness of cohort studies is that you can never be entirely sure about cause and effect. If, for example, you discover that people who eat a Mediterranean diet live longer, is that really just because of the diet or could it be that the people who eat that way also do more exercise and are more health conscious? The researchers try to allow for these other factors, but can never be sure they are really are comparing like with like.

That's why it's so important to also do randomized controlled trials—where you get a group of people and then randomly allocate them to treatment A or treatment B and follow them over time to see what happens. I have mentioned randomized controlled trials quite a bit in this book.

Further Measurements and Tests

The following tests are useful but not essential. You may be able to get some or all of them free on the NHS.

Blood pressure—High blood pressure puts you at greater risk of heart disease and stroke. The Fast800 will bring your blood pressure down. Fast. If you are currently on blood pressure medication you will need to talk to your doctor about reducing the medication, because you don't want it to fall too low.

A1c—This measures glycated hemoglobin and gives an overall picture of what your average blood sugar levels have been like over the previous 2–3 months.

LFTs—Liver function tests can show if you have unhealthy levels of fat in your liver as this causes liver inflammation with raised liver enzymes. The Fast800 is very effective at reducing liver fat.

Lipids—This is a test looking at your cholesterol profile. It will give you an idea of your risk of stroke or heart disease and usually improves on the Fast800.

U&Es—This measures the salts in your blood and is an indicator of how well your kidneys are functioning. Being overweight or having diabetes can lead to significant kidney problems.

Full blood count—This will show if you are within the normal range.

Thyroid Function Tests (TFTs)—The thyroid is a gland that sits in front of the neck and helps to control metabolism. If this is underactive you will feel tired and put on weight easily. If you think you have an underactive thyroid it may be worth having your TFTs checked prior to starting a diet program to ensure that it's not contributing to your problems.

Measuring your levels of insulin and insulin resistance

I've written a lot about the dangers of having high levels of insulin and being insulin resistant. These are not standard tests, but you can arrange to have them done privately.

Measuring your visceral (tummy) fat levels

As well as measuring your waist, you might want to get a DEXA scan. A DEXA (Dual Energy X-ray Absorptiometry) scan is a full-body, low-dose X-ray scan that accurately measures fat and muscle, as well as bone density.

If, like me, you are a TOFI (Thin on the Outside, Fat Inside), it will reveal how much visceral fat you have. This should fall rapidly in the first few weeks of the Fast800.

NOTES

1. www.nhs.uk/live-well/healthy-weight/top-diets-review/.
2. Trends in U.S. Per Capita Consumption of Dairy Products, 1970-2012. USDA, 2014. www.ers.usda.gov/amber-waves/2014/june/trends-in-us-per-capita-consumption-of-dairy-products-1970-2012/.

   Gross L, Li Li et al., "Increased Consumption of Refined Carbohydrates and the Epidemic of Type 2 Diabetes in the United States: An Ecologic Assessment." *Amer J Clin Nutr*, 2004. https://academic.oup.com/ajcn/article/79/5/774/4690186.
3. *New York Times*, "Always Hungry? Here's Why."
4. Trends in U.S. Per Capita Consumption of Dairy Products, 1970–2012. USDA, 2014. www.ers.usda.gov/amber-waves/2014/june/trends-in-us-per-capita-consumption-of-dairy-products-1970-2012/.
5. "Which Foods May Be Addictive?" https://journals.plos.org/plosone/article?id=10.1371/journal.pone.0117959.
6. www.crsociety.org/index.html.
7. Fabien Pifferi et al., "Caloric Restriction Increases Lifespan But Affects Brain Integrity in Grey Mouse Lemur Primates." *Communications Biology*, 2018 DOI: 10.1038/s42003-018-0024-8.
8. Valter D. Longo et al., "Prolonged Fasting Reduces IGF-1/PKA to Promote Hematopoietic-Stem-Cell-Based Regeneration and Reverse Immunosuppression." *Cell Stem Cell*, 2014; 14 (6).

9. www.thetimes.co.uk/article/eat-less-live-longer-the-diet -that-holds-the-key-to-staying-young-2t662n633).

10. Carter S, Clifton PM, and Keogh JB., "Effect of Intermittent Compared With Continuous Energy Restricted Diet on Glycemic Control in Patients With Type 2 Diabetes." *Diabetes Res Clin Pract*, 2016. www.ncbi.nlm.nih.gov/pubmed/27833048.

11. Harvie M, Wright C et al., "The Effect of Intermittent Energy and Carbohydrate Restriction V. Daily Energy Restriction on Weight Loss and Metabolic Disease Risk Markers in Overweight Women." *Br J Nutr*, 2013. www.ncbi.nlm.nih .gov/pubmed/23591120.

12. Harvie M, Sims AH et al., "Intermittent Energy Restriction Induces Changes in Breast Gene Expression and Systemic Metabolism." *Breast Cancer Res.*, 2016. www.ncbi.nlm.nih.gov /pubmed/27233359.

13. Antoni R, Johnston KL et al., "Intermittent V. Continuous Energy Restriction: Differential Effects on Postprandial Glucose and Lipid Metabolism Following Matched Weight Loss in Overweight/Obese Participants." *Br J Nutr*, 2018. www.ncbi .nlm.nih.gov/pubmed/29508693.

14. Megumi Hatori, Christopher Vollmers et al., "Time Restricted Feeding Without Reducing Caloric Intake Prevents Metabolic Diseases in Mice Fed a High Fat Diet." *Cell Metab*, 2012. www.ncbi.nlm.nih.gov/pmc/articles/PMC3491655.

15. Antoni R, Robertson TM et al., "A Pilot Feasibility Study Exploring the Effects of a Moderate Time-Restricted Feeding Intervention on Energy Intake, Adiposity and Metabolic Physiology in Free-Living Human Subjects." www.cambridge .org/core/services/aop-cambridge-core/content/view/S204867 9018000137.

16. Gabel K, Hoddy K et al., "Effects of 8-Hour Time Restricted Feeding on Body Weight and Metabolic Disease Risk Factors in Obese Adults: A Pilot Study." *Nutr. Healthy Aging*,

2018. https://www.ncbi.nlm.nih.gov/pmc/articles/PMC600 4924/#!po=0.724638.

17. Pierce JP, Faerber S et al., "The Women's Healthy Eating and Living (WHEL)," 2016.

18. Taylor R, Lean M. DiRECT (Diabetes Remission Clinical Trial), 2017. www.ncl.ac.uk/press/articles/archive/2017/12 /directstudy/.

19. Rogelholm M, Larsen TM et al., "PREVention of Diabetes Through Lifestyle Intervention and Population Studies in Europe and Around the World." *Nutrients*, 2017. www.ncbi.nlm .nih.gov/pubmed/28632180.

20. Jebb S, Astbury N et al., "Doctor Referral of Overweight People to a Low-Energy Treatment (DROPLET) in primary care using total diet replacement products." bmjopen.bmj .com/content/7/8/e016709.

21. Purcell K, Sumithran P et al., "The Effect of Rate of Weight Loss on Long-Term Weight Management: A Randomised Controlled Trial." *Lancet Diabetes Endocrinol*, 2014. www.ncbi.nlm.nih.gov/pubmed/25459211.

22. Keys A et al., *The Biology of Human Starvation* (2 vols). Oxford, England: Univ. of Minnesota Press, 1950. http://psyc net.apa.org/record/1951-02195-000.

23. Zauner C, Schneeweiss B et al., "Resting Energy Expenditure in Short-Term Starvation is Increased as A Result of an Increase in Serum Norepinephrine." *Am J Clin Nutr*, 2000. www.ncbi.nlm.nih.gov/pubmed/10837292.

24. Gomez-Arbelaez D, Crujeiras AB et al., Resting Metabolic Rate of Obese Patients Under Very Low Calorie Ketogenic Diet. *Nutr Metab*, 2018. www.ncbi.nlm.nih.gov/pmc/articles /PMC5816424.

25. Taylor R, Lean M. DiRECT (Diabetes Remission Clinical Trial), 2017. https://www.ncl.ac.uk/press/articles/archive/2017 /12/directstudy/.

26. Schor J., "Prevención con Dieta Mediterránea." *Nat Med J*, 2015. www.naturalmedicinejournal.com/journal/2015-02 /prevenci%C3%B3n-con-dieta-mediterr%C3%A1nea-cohort -2-years-later.

27. Lassale C, Batty GD et al., "Healthy Dietary Indices and Risk of Depressive Outcomes: A Systematic Review and Meta-Analysis of Observational Studies." *Molecular Psychiatry*, 2018. www.nature.com/articles/s41380-018-0237-8.

28. Shai I, Schwarzfuchs D et al., "Weight Loss with a Low-Carbohydrate, Mediterranean, or Low-Fat Diet." *N Engl J Med*, 2008. www.nejm.org/doi/full/10.1056/NEJMoa0708681.

29. Gepner Y, Shelef I et al., "Effect of Distinct Lifestyle Interventions on Mobilization of Fat Storage Pools: CENTRAL Magnetic Resonance Imaging Randomized Controlled Trial." *Circulation*, 2018.

30. Jakicic JM, Davis KK et al., "Effect of Wearable Technology Combined With a Lifestyle Intervention on Long-term Weight Loss." *JAMA*, 2016. www.ncbi.nlm.nih.gov/pubmed /27654602.

31. Gillen JB, Martin BJ et al., "Twelve Weeks of Sprint Interval Training Improves Indices of Cardiometabolic Health Similar to Traditional Endurance Training despite a Five-Fold Lower Exercise Volume and Time Commitment." *PLOS One*, 2016. www.ncbi.nlm.nih.gov/pubmed/27115 137/.

32. Khatib HK et al., "The Effects of Partial Sleep Deprivation on Energy Balance." *EJCN*, 2016. www.nature.com/articles /ejcn2016201.

33. Jacka F, O'Neil A et al., "A Randomised Controlled Trial of Dietary Improvement for Adults With Major Depression (the 'SMILES' trial)." *BMC Medicine*, 2017. bmcmedicine.biomed central.com/articles/10.1186/s12916-017-0791-y.

34. Byrne NM, Sainsbury A et al., "Minimising Adaptive

Thermogenesis and Deactivating Obesity Rebound." *Intern Jnl of Obesity*, 2017. www.nature.com/articles/ijo2017206.

35. Moro T, Tinsley G et al., "Effects of Eight Weeks of Time-Restricted Feeding (16/8) on Basal Metabolism, Maximal Strength, Body Composition, Inflammation, and Cardiovascular Risk Factors in Resistance-Trained Males." *Jnl of Translational Med*, 2016. https://translational-medicine.bio medcentral.com/articles/10.1186/s12967-016-1044-0.

36. VanWormer J, Linde JA et al., "Self-Weighing Frequency is Associated with Weight Gain Prevention over Two Years among Working Adults." *Int. J. Behav. Med.*, 2012. www.ncbi .nlm.nih.gov/pmc/articles/PMC3474347/.

37. Poncela-Casasnovas J, Spring B et al., "Social Embeddedness in An Online Weight Management Program is Linked to Greater Weight Loss." *J R Soc Interface*, 2015. www.ncbi.nlm .nih.gov/pubmed/25631561.

38. Gorin A, Phelan S et al., "Involving Support Partners in Obesity Treatment." *J. Consult Clin Psychol*, 2005. www.ncbi .nlm.nih.gov/pubmed/15796642.

39. Carriere K, Khoury B et al., "Mindfulness-Based Interventions for Weight Loss: A Systematic Review and Meta-Analysis." *Obes Rev*, 2018. www.ncbi.nlm.nih.gov/pubmed/29076610.

40. "Kaiser Permanente Study Finds Keeping a Food Diary Doubles Diet Weight Loss." *Amer J Prev Med*, 2008. https:// share.kaiserpermanente.org/article/kaiser-permanente-study -finds-keeping-a-food-diary-doubles-diet-weight-loss/.

41. Poole R, Kennedy O et al., "Coffee Consumption and Health: Umbrella Review of Meta-Analyses of Multiple Health Outcomes." *BMJ*, 2017. www.bmj.com/content/359/bmj.j5024.

42. Health Professionals Follow-up Study. https://sites.sph .harvard.edu/hpfs/.

INDEX

Dr. Michael Mosley is a science presenter, journalist, and executive producer. After training to be a doctor at the Royal Free Hospital in London, he spent 25 years at the BBC, where he made numerous science documentaries. Now freelance, he is the author of several bestselling books, *The FastDiet*, *The 8-Week Blood Sugar Diet*, and *The Clever Gut Diet*. He is married with four children. Please visit thefast800.com for more information.

Dr. Clare Bailey, wife of Michael Mosley, is a general practitioner who has pioneered a dietary approach to health and reducing blood sugars and diabetes at her practice in Buckinghamshire. She is the author of *The 8-Week Blood Sugar Diet Cookbook* and *The Clever Gut Diet Cookbook*.